Remove the Thorn
and
GOD Will Heal

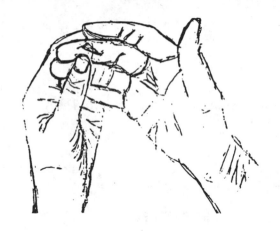

By

BUD CURTIS

BELCO
WHITTIER, CALIFORNIA

REMOVE THE THORN AND GOD WILL HEAL

Dedication

This book is dedicated to God, in thanks for His Son, the Lord Jesus Christ, and the Holy Spirit for helping me to find wisdom and knowledge, and for opening doors that enabled me to succeed with the research revealed in this book.

Contents

Foreword

It is with great pleasure that I was asked to write a Foreword to a book by Bud Curtis. He has dedicated himself to life-building programs and to people who want to live life on the higher road. It is the higher road in life in which I've always been interested. We all deserve the very best.

Very few of us care to assure that we always make the choices that serve our bodies best. It is time that people recognize that we cannot serve our bodies through proper nutrition alone, although proper nutrition is essential to good health. Neither can we serve our body just through mechanical arts. And it goes without saying that we cannot allow coffee and doughnuts and junk foods to circulate around in our systems.

It is time that we consider good nutrition for

both physical and spiritual aspects of our beings. In order to keep our bodies well, it takes the proper amount of spiritual, mental, emotional, physical, chemical, and mechanical efforts. We cannot have a good body unless it is considered from a wholistic standpoint. To live on Coca-Cola on one hand and to pray with the other is not consistent with the higher laws of life. If we're going to do the right thing in one direction, we can do it in all directions.

However, I feel that one of the greatest things that's going to come about one of these days is that we're going to sit down and work this out from the spiritual standpoint first, and then, as the next logical step, we'll take care of the physical. The physical things usually are easy to do . . . if we want to do them and have a love for doing them. We must have a love for what we *have to do* in this life. That is not the same as always doing the things we love to do; it is loving the things that we *must* do in life. We must take care of our physical body to have a good physical existence, but our leadership comes from the spiritual side of life. The spiritual side of life will lead us into accepting that which is good for us . . . in our education, our schools, our home, our marriage, our job, or in whatever efforts that we may be putting into life.

It is to this end that we realize that our endeavors in life are the only thing by which we can be measured at the end of our lives. By that we will be judged. It is well that we grasp this important concept—we need spiritual leadership for the physical things of this body. The needs follow the spiritual and mental things. The lungs breathe according to the spiritual aspect. We are relieved, we believe, and we carry on because of motivation, inspiration, and aspirations.

And to this end, recognizing that Bud Curtis brings out so much vital information in his book concerning the spiritual, mental, and physical aspects of life, that it gives me great pleasure to add these words of commendation for his efforts in helping people. Going the healing way is necessary for the future. We have had enough treatments, enough of taking care of only the physical. It is now that we look to the wholistic art—caring for the person spirit, soul, and body—so that whatever we do, we have the approval of God.

Who satisfied thy mouth with good things; so that thy youth is renewed like the eagle's. Psalms 103:5

The Lord is the Spirit who gives them life, and where He is there is freedom [from trying to be saved by keeping the laws of God].
II Corinthians 3:17 (The Living Bible)

Dr. Bernard Jensen
Escondidio, California
May 1993

Acknowledgments

Special thanks to my wife
Winona
for helping me and for all the time she allowed
me to spend in research accumulating the
evidence needed to enable me to write
this book, so mankind may clean his
body and make it a fit dwelling place
. . . a temple of God, so that all
disease goes away.
Also to
Jim Spillman
for the prepublication review of this
book for Scriptural accuracy
and to
Julie Hepner,
Don McAlvany,
and Lindsey Williams
for their enthusiastic testimonials.

About the Author—
Bud Curtis

I was born in a small town in Texas. We were a poor family, but we were able to survive. In fact the entire area was poor, but in these little towns the folks were happy.

I tried to get ahead in that part of the country, but with little success. Therefore, like so many others, I moved to California and went into business for myself. My company was involved in the aerospace industry, building environmental control systems for military fighters, including being a prime contractor for the U.S. Air Force.

After nearly 25 years in the business, I retired from the same position where I started...I just couldn't figure out how to get promoted! I guess when you start at the top, you end up at the top.

I sold the company, but like so many other

people, while I was in the business of accumulating wealth, I paid little attention to my lifestyle, and gradually lost my health. It is typical for entrepreneurs to get wrapped up in fighting the battle of making money and becoming successful and to destroy their bodies in the process. I was one of those "typical" people. Even though I was only 45 when I retired, I had all the aches and pains and illnesses that go along with neglecting one's body for that many years. However, since I was so young, I decided to go in search of a way to get my health back.

I sought out many doctors and listened to endless lectures and read more books and articles than a librarian. In 1956, I went to Dr. Bernard Jensen's ranch, and after he had examined me, he told me a number of things I should do (or stop doing). I tried some of them, with little or no effort . . . and, therefore, little or no effect. I was not convinced his advice was correct, and I was still looking for the "magic pill" to take. So I continued my search and met many world renowned doctors, attended thousands of lectures, and read more books. I didn't find my "magic pill," but each one gave me a hunger for more knowledge in this area, so I prayed for healing, wisdom, and knowledge.

I received wisdom and knowledge, however, with regard to healing of diseases, what I encountered were many, many doctors who told me that the only disease we have is toxemia (or autointoxication, which means that we are toxic inside our own body . . . in other words, our systems are all plugged up with toxins, so nothing functions properly). One day a doctor said to me, "When you hurt enough, you'll do what is necessary to get well." So I tried the tissue cleansing described in the book by Dr. Jensen, and it helped; I tried vitamins, I tried minerals, I tried juices, and they all helped . . . but it was a *real inconvenience*. It just took more time than I was willing to give at that point—I was still hoping for that "magic pill."

Later, I became involved with the clinics and hospitals in Mexico. I even referred some of my friends there, and they were in much worse health than I was. They got better but a strange thing would happen. They'd be fine for a few years, but a different disease would come upon them, or the same disease would return, perhaps in a different part of the body. The more I got involved in Mexico trying to find out which clinic had the "magic pill," the more evident one fact became over a period of several years. I finally realized, by getting involved in some of the blood workups at the clinics, how you could orchestrate the body with herbs, nutrition, and medicine. It was fascinating. However, I noticed one thing in common with all of the people: how toxic their bowels and livers were, which led me to the cleansing of the colon and the blood, and subsequently to the other tissues of the body.

In trying to make my body the temple of God, as we are instructed in I Corinthians 3:16, I was convinced that I should do my very best to remove the problems, so my body would have a chance to heal. That is what led me to the research for this book. As each of us is a "cell" or "member" in the body of Christ, I want *my* cell to be clean and functioning properly—spiritually and physically—so that I don't pull down my brother or sister because of my own poor health or disease.

My prayers are with you, and I hope you will take an interest in your bodies and follow some of the suggestions indicated by the research that I have done.

Your author,

Bud

Introduction

Some of you are waiting for God to heal your aches, pains, and diseases. I encourage you to start cleansing your body so healing can take place. Then, ask God for His help in restoring your body to good health.

Many of you already have used this program and found it to work, and many have written letters and testimonials about their healing (some are included in this book). For this, all praise and glory to Jesus.

There is great need among the members of the Body of Christ for ongoing health. Because of environmental conditions and the things we have been putting into our bodies (in the name of food), many believers suffer a myriad of conditions need-lessly. . .conditions that hinder their ability to serve the Lord as they desire to in their hearts.

The Word tells us that God's people perish for a lack of knowledge (Hosea 4:6). If we lack spiritual knowledge, we perish spiritually; if we lack knowledge of how to properly maintain our physical frames, they, too, will perish. What we must recognize is that there is no excuse for the lack of either type of knowledge; the Word of God is replete with information and instruction of both a spiritual and physical nature.

We are asked, "Know you not that your bodies are the temple of the Holy Spirit?" Well, as a courtesy to Him who indwells the believer's body, with the side benefit of the good health that we may enjoy, should we not attempt to provide a clean "temple" for Him?

In this book, we try to enlighten you first about the seriousness of this subject, then we show you the problem areas and how they became a problem to our health, and finally, we show you how you can do something about it... in a very practical, down-to-earth plan which anyone can put into practice to cleanse his/her body and maintain it in that state.

Pastors, elders, and spiritual leaders, I particularly want to emphasize the importance of you being cleansed physically, as well as spiritually. You are the under-shepherds of God's flocks, placed in leadership by the spiritual gifts given to you by our Lord. It is part of your responsibility to set good examples for those in your care. Remember, Paul told the people in one local church that they should follow him, as he followed Christ. That didn't mean that he had set himself up as another "mediator" between them and Jesus; it merely meant that he was living out an example of how they should live their daily lives. As water seeks its own level, the people will not rise above their leadership, especially when it is something that involves personal discipline and learning new patterns for daily living.

It is a verified truth that *we are what we eat.* Unfortunately, for the sake of convenience, and frequently because we felt we had no other choice, we have dropped most of our standards regarding our food intake. Our diets consist mainly of fast foods, highly processed foods, junk foods, and foods lacking in nutrition or full of antibiotics and pesticides because of the way they were grown. *Please note: There are options!* I trust the things you learn in this book will prove beneficial to you. . . spirit, soul, and body.

Each promise of God is available to each child of God, however, they are always conditional; that is, they are "if. . .then" promises. For example, "if we confess our sins". . . "He is faithful and just to forgive our sins." "Believe on the Lord Jesus Christ". . . "And thou shalt be saved." He has promised "when two or three gather in My name" . . . "There am I in the midst." "If you believe in your heart and doubt not,"—there are several important scriptures that begin this way and end with a number of different promises, such as "ask anything in My name," "tell the mountain to be cast into the sea, and it shall be done," "whatsoever you say," and others, but the majority of them end the same way . . . "That the Father may be glorified in the Son." The fact that there are conditions with each promise doesn't mean that we can earn these promises by our works; it is still through the grace of God that we receive any of the many promises in the Word. However, we also are told that "obedience is better than sacrifice," and I like to think of these as "instructions" from God (because He knows better than we do what is good for us) followed by a blessing for obedience. First, we must get our own house in order—spiritually and physically—if we are to be effective witnesses, and once we have done so, start spreading the news . . . the rest of the world needs it as badly as we do!

Unlike so many other religions, we do not have to guess what it takes to please our God. Our God loves us, and He clearly spells out everything in His Word, so we know exactly *what* to obey, and because He is faithful and He cannot lie, we know that He will keep His part of the promise, if we keep ours. I want to leave you with four scriptures as we move into chapter one. And may all that is said in the following pages only bring glory to the Father, through Jesus, the Son.

For if there be first a willing mind. . . .
II Corinthians 8:12

For with God nothing shall be impossible.
Luke 1:37

. . . *"If thou wilt diligently hearken to the voice of the Lord thy God, and wilt do that which is right in His sight, and wilt give ear to His commandments, and keep all his statutes, I will put none of these diseases upon thee, . . . for I am the Lord that healeth thee."*   Exodus 15:26

Bless the Lord, O my soul, and forget not all his benefits; . . . who healeth all thy diseases; . . . .   Psalms 103:2,3

Chapter 1

Help, Lord!
We Lost Our Canopy

It is probable that at the beginning of the earth, God created a protective moisture barrier which reached several miles out into the stratosphere. The environment was like a small mist at all times. The oxygen content, because of the moisture barrier around the earth, was much greater than today...up to 21% to 22%—today the best you can have is about 14.7%.

Because of the high oxygen content of the earth at that time, and because of the moisture that was in the canopy, it was an ideal environment for rapid and lush growth. Because this canopy would produce a "greenhouse" type of environment, you can predict that there was a universally warm temperature in which everything would grow in great abundance. A higher oxygen content would make vegetation grow faster and bigger.

According to the Bible (Genesis 5:5), many men before the Flood of Noah lived to be around 900 to 1,000 years old. Noah lived to be 950 years old; Adam lived to be 930 years old; and Methuselah actually lived to be 969 years old. Because of the excellent environment in which they lived—without any pollution and protected by their canopy from the effect of ultraviolet rays—every normal breath of air that they took would be equivalent to a *deep* breath for us. And because there was so much more oxygen in their air, with every breath they took, they got a lot more oxygen into their bloodstream than we can.

Now, if you hiked up to the tall mountains, say 10,000 or 12,000 feet, where the oxygen is thinner, you would have to breathe a lot more than at a lower altitude. So you would be struggling all the time, perhaps panting like a dog trying to get enough oxygen into your lungs to supply your body. Before the canopy fell, at the Flood, this was not the case. Now, however, we must be aware of our need for more oxygen intake and make a conscious effort to breathe very deeply on a regular basis. You would be surprised at how much more alert you would be if you would do even that much. But it is an effort, and we tend to be relaxed in what we do, so we don't breathe as deeply as we should. But deep breathing from time to time would bring great benefits to your body, especially during long stretches of concentration at your work, or driving, for example.

Now, Noah, when he was running around building the Ark, kept telling those people it was going to rain, but they laughed at him because they didn't know what rain was. The Bible tells us that before the Flood the earth was watered with a dew that came up from the earth. This was a condition created by the canopy. But when it did start to rain, for 40 days and nights—you know the story—the Lord had the canopy fall, which along with the fountains of the deep (underwater volcanic activity) provided the water necessary to cover the globe. Mankind, land animals, and plants were destroyed, except for those on the Ark with Noah. God gave them a chance to start anew, including the earth itself; but even though the plants did grow again after nearly a year under water, it was a much harsher environment, with much less vegetation, and no canopy for protection or abundant oxygen.

I do not believe there were any temperature extremes in the Garden of Eden. They had exactly the right temperature for man to grow and be prosperous. The soil that produced the fruits and vegetables was perfect, because God had made it and proclaimed it "very good." The food was perfect, as well, and it had a high content of oxygen. Because of this, there was no disease as we know it, no viruses, harmful bacteria, fermentation, or fungus.

In order for something to decay, it has to fall on the ground, then the chemical reaction would start it decaying. But any fruit that was on the tree would not become over-ripe or rotten. Because of the high oxygen content, it was impossible to have fermentation. That was proven to my satisfaction when I read in Genesis 9:20,21 about Noah's first vineyard after the Flood. When he harvested the grapes, he did as he always had . . . squeezed the grapes to make the juice, but this particular time he got drunk (the text implies he was not expecting that result), so Noah was "privileged" to be the first drunk recorded in the Bible.

Now, when there is fermentation, it actually takes oxygen out of the product. Fermentation occurs because of the yeast and sugar content of the grapes (or any other food), and today we can have all the fermentation we want. Of course, if there were no fermentation, it would be impossible to make wine, alcohol, cigarettes, narcotics, and a few of those things we don't really need in this world, anyway. In many cases, people actually are fermenting their own flesh inside their own bodies. Because of toxins and fermentation of the starches that they eat, and the sugar content, they actually are creating fermentation at the cellular level of the body. We will discuss that more in the section on cleansing, chapter five.

But we find that in God's design for mankind, He gave us oxygen, which is O_2—2 atoms of oxygen—exactly what man needed to sustain life. Without the oxygen, we can't survive very many minutes. We can go many days without food, we can go quite some time without water, but man cannot go very long without oxygen. If you were with someone right now who was having a heart attack, the first thing you would give them would be oxygen. If you were drunk, the first thing they would give you to keep you from being intoxicated would be oxygen. In my opinion, oxygen is the "wonder drug" that God gave us. We misuse it, abuse it, and contaminate it, but still it was God-given and to me it is the very entity of life. When God speaks of breathing in life, oxygen is the breath of life.

In addition to tremendous amounts of vegetation because of the oxygen, moisture, and mild climate provided by the pre-Flood canopy, the canopy also allowed animals to grow to great size. Whether or not we believe the alleged "prehistoric" animals were there (dinosaurs and flying reptiles, for example), they weren't necessarily in the Garden of Eden (although there is no indication in the Bible of creatures being brought into existence anywhere else, and God did pass them all before Adam and have him name them (Gen. 2:19,20), so it is reasonable to assume that they may have been in the garden). They could have been in other regions of the earth—we know from excavation that plant life was prolific at the north and south poles at one time in history. The majority of them were herbivorous (in fact, they all probably were prior to the Flood), and the greenhouse effect produced by the canopy most assuredly would have provided sufficient vegetation to sustain them. Noah had plenty of room on the Ark to have accommodated them, therefore, in all probability the lack of the canopy and the lack of the lush vegetation produced by it (their food) probably was a major contributing factor in their extinction. Only God knows for sure if these oversized crea- tures lived contemporaneously with man, but the evidence geologists are finding lately seems to be pointing in that direction, most notably the fossil prints in the bed of the Paluxy River in Glen Rose, Texas. And of course, we have the scriptural refer- ences in Job to behemoth and dragons, and his- torical legends about dragons from all around the globe...legends that still survive to this day.

But if, in fact, they did exist with man, the reason they could grow to such gigantic proportions was because of the food chain they were eating. They had an abundance of food, just like man had an abundance of food because. And while they were still in the Garden (prior to the fall), mankind was not required to obtain his food by the "sweat of his brow," except, of course, for bread.

In order to have bread, you have to grind the grain and bake the bread. Other than that, they just picked it off the tree and ate it. I believe man messes up everything he touches, but this particu- lar time, it was a big mess-up. And if you accept the canopy theory, you can see how far we have degenerated from a perfect world, perfect in oxy- gen, moisture, and food...and perfect in relation to God. Imagine a relationship so perfect that God would come down every day and walk with them in the cool of the evening. Now we not only have to earn our living by the sweat of our brow, we literally have to struggle with each breath to take in enough life-sustaining oxygen to provide the fuel needed by every cell in our bodies. The cells in your body use oxygen as fuel—they don't use food as fuel.

So, oxygen is the fuel for man, and because we no longer have a high concentration of oxygen in either our food or our air, our bodies are suffering. What your body needs is enough oxygen to completely oxidize each and every cell in your body. It needs a clean, free-flowing output of blood, carrying lots of oxygen to every cell of your body, as well as the nutrition, and the waste to be carried away from each cell. That's exactly the way God designed our bodies.

If we did exactly what we should do in order to be good stewards, making our bodies perfect temples for God (I Cor. 3:16,17; 6:19; II Cor. 6:16; Eph. 3:33), we would be much better able to do the Lord's work. Back before the Flood, it was much easier. But today we are having more trouble, so the diet on which we live should be rich in oxygen, because oxygen could help us to benefit, reform, and rebuild each and every cell in our bodies.

I've heard that in Gary, Indiana, a couple of years ago—because of the electric furnaces of the steel mills around Gary—instead of the oxygen content being 14.7%, it was down below 8%. People were dropping on the streets, passing out, having to go to the hospital because of the low oxygen environment created by the pollution in that particular town. The more we pollute, the less oxygen we have.

Remember those animals living in the ocean, such as the whales? They don't experience the same suffering we do, furthermore, they still live relatively long lifespans, because they get their oxygen from the water, not from the atmosphere. I'm sure there must be less oxygen in the water than there was many years ago. Oxygen gets into the ocean water from the photosynthesis of plankton that grows in the sea, which puts oxygen into the water through the process of algae growing. If you look very closely at a lake—any lake that's healthy—on a real still day you can see tiny little bubbles coming to the surface, and you'll notice those tiny little bubbles are always over the top of where plants and grass and green items are growing at the bottom of the lake. That's what's putting oxygen into the water. It's the same with the plankton in the ocean. Therefore, the whales and the sea animals that breath in the water and get their oxygen from the water do not experience the same difficulties that we do. Some of them, like the turtles, still live to great ages.

Your brain needs 20% of the oxygen that you breathe, but it's only 2% of the weight of your body. A lot of people are walking around today feeling tired, unable to function in their mind, unable to perform to the benefit of their job because of lack of sufficient oxygen to the brain.

I challenge you to do an exercise right now that costs you nothing. If you'll do this correctly, you'll find that you are much more alert and that you feel better. And it only takes a couple of minutes.

The best thing to do is either stand up or sit erect and take four deep breaths, as deep as you can, do not hold them—just breathe them in and let them out. You don't have to do it fast, but take as deep a breath as you can. After doing the first four, you may notice a "head rush" coming up through your neck into your head; immediately take four more deep ones. Some of you may feel like you're going to pass out. I doubt if you would, because it's oxygen that's getting into your brain, and the brain is suffering all the time from of lack of oxygen.

So, take the eight deep breaths, and if you could, every breath the rest of your life. If you would deep breathe, you not only would feel better, you would react better, think better, and have a better attitude toward life. At least do it every hour or half hour. Just try it a few times and see if your life doesn't improve . . . just from increasing the amount of oxygen that's going to your brain. Give your brain a chance. It's like having a beautiful computer, then turning off the power, at least turning off half the power so the computer can't work. Give your computer a chance—your brain—and let's see if we can't get a little bit more alert, so we can do a little bit better job.

Chapter 2

How to Pollute Your Body Without Even Trying

Pollution! Is it just the smog in Los Angeles, or the rivers full of toxic waste in the big industrial states? Not so! The world is full of pollution since the fall of man, and it is growing worse rapidly since the loss of our canopy; then came the industrial revolution and the concentration of the population into localized regions. Thereafter, the pollution began to increase exponentially.

Then we deliberately began to add to the pollution by putting all sorts of chemical (unnatural) additives into our soil and on our plants, and later, even into our drinking water...herbicides, insecticides, pesticides, fertilizers, chlorine, fluoride, bromines, etc. (Of course, the additives to the water were necessitated by our mistreatment of the land and environment, which we earlier had contaminated, and it subsequently reached our water supply.)

Now, as much as I would like to tell you otherwise, unfortunately, there is no way for all this pollution NOT to get into man's food chain, as well as into the air which he breathes. In other words, *we pollute our bodies without even trying*—if we live on planet earth today, it is just unavoidable. In fact, even when we try with great resolve to eliminate toxic substances from our air and food, it is not totally possible, even if we are willing to make a great lifestyle change.

Toxins! If there is one thing I want you to understand and remember from this book, it is this: Illness is just a symptom; it is not the disease. The *true* disease is *toxemia,* or to put it simply, a toxin-permeated, unclean body, which—in its weakened state—is unable to defend itself against certain physical attacks. These manifest themselves by any number of different "labels," but have one cause . . . an unhealthy, toxin-laden body. Later in this book we will address what you can do to rid your body of these toxins and regain your health (see Chapter 5). But for now, I want to address some of the specific areas of pollution and what we can do to help alleviate them.

These are some of the everyday problems that I think are in the everyday life of the average person.

Water

One of the major problems is the water . . . both the water you drink and the water in which you bathe. Many people, especially those in the large metropolitan areas who are drinking city water right out of the tap, think the sollution to their drinking water problem is to buy bottled water. But it has been proven in testing that the bottled water you are buying, in most cases, is not fit for consumption.

Most bottlers simply take the city water and filter it, then add flavor to it (or treat it in some way) to try to make it drinkable, so you do not smell the pollution (or the chlorine or other additives they use to try and make it safe to drink). I doubt seriously that of the 700 different brands of bottled water on the market that you would find a very large percentage actually fit to drink, if you sent the water out to an independent laboratory and had it analyzed. The problem is that it has too much pollution from the ground, from the air, and from the waste from the landfills, which seep down into the aquifers (the underground water table), contaminating them heavily with harmful chemicals of all types, destroying our water systems.

A law has been passed by the federal government that all municipal water systems must treat their water with chlorine. Chlorine is one of the very deadliest chemicals. However, it is not only the chlorine gas or the chlorine chemical that it so harmful, it is what it kills. Chlorine is supposed to kill the bad bugs in the water, the bacteria, the viruses, etc. Well, if it will kill the bad ones, it will also kill the good ones. Therefore, if you are drinking chlorinated water, you also are destroying the good bacteria that are in your body, and if you are doing that, you will have an awfully hard time ever balancing your system.

Purifying the Water

The only way to make this water really safe to drink is to mechanically clean it by putting it through a system to remove the additives and impurities. But the question is, "What kind of system?" The market is flooded with every imaginable type of water treatment system, and I am going to give you the benefit of my personal experience in this matter.

First, let's discuss the "filter" systems. I know a lot of people buy these special filtering systems that "filter this and filter that," and you'll hear some of them say that they filter out the viruses, and the bacteria, and the algae, and the herbicides. Well, I'm sorry to say that that's not possible. The best filter that's known to mankind is only a half micron, and yet a virus is 1/20th of one micron. So how could a filter possibly filter out a virus? It may filter out some of the large bacteria, but I have doubts about that.

Some companies will tell you that their product contains a special silver coating that will kill the "varmints." Well, I'm sorry, but I don't believe that either. What I might believe is that in some cases people are selling you reverse osmosis (RO) units, which are good. However, I found out that the storage tank (only about three gallons) that came with the reverse osmosis unit I had in my own house was permitting bacteria to form in it because it had a rubber bladder.

I understand that England now has outlawed all RO systems, unless they contain a double-pass UV method. As the water goes into the storage tank it is treated by ultraviolet light, and again when it comes out it is treated by ultraviolet light. Then it can be delivered to your tap without any bacteria or viruses that are harmful to you. Exception: in some cases you may get the "ghost effect." If in your water you have some large particles, for example, calcium or magnesium, and these particles are large enough for a bacteria to ride "piggyback" on the opposite side of the particle as it passes through the UV, it won't be killed, so you'll still be drinking it.

However, if you have a double-pass UV on your RO system, you probably have a fairly decent system for purifying the water in your home.

The ionized filtration, distillation. . . all of these have some merit, but here is the fairly simple system that I use: A simple four-stage pre-filter, an RO system with at least a single-, but preferably a double-pass UV, and then a four-stage post-filter, because some of the filters now have things in them that help take out metals.

As a further step, after it comes out of our

storage tank, it goes into a container which we treat with activated oxygen. We bubble activated oxygen into the water for at least three minutes. We feel that whatever our filters, RO system, UV, and charcoal might miss will be finished off by the activated oxygen (ozone).

Also, putting oxygen back into the water makes it taste more like mountain spring water. When you taste that water from the mountain stream, bubbling down right through the high Sierras or some high mountain range, it tastes good. And the reason it tastes good is because of the dissolved oxygen. It's not the minerals that are in the water; minerals have little or no flavor. What you are trying to achieve is getting as much oxygen into the water as it will accept. What happens as it passes down this mountain stream is that it saturates itself with the maximum amount of dissolved oxygen that it possibly can assimilate. And that's what you really want—that's what God meant for us to drink. That's what would help us to be healthy.

Then, of course, all the good filtration systems are charcoal in the last filtration stage, because charcoal does a better job of cleansing. But (depending upon your water) in some cases the charcoal becomes polluted in such a short period of time that it also contributes to the process of creating bacteria (because it becomes so contaminated). However, when used in conjunction with the UV *before* it goes through the charcoal, it actually has a tendency to clean the charcoal, rather than pollute it. So that's my personal preference.

Chlorine Absorption

Now, I would like to share with you some startling documented facts about the absorption of chemicals. The skin is so efficient at absorption, that your intake of chemicals is much higher when bathing or swimming in them, than when you ingest them orally. Please study carefully the following report on some important research:

SKIN ABSORPTION

Preliminary research suggests that the ingestion of harmful chemicals from drinking water may not be the primary route of exposure. Both skin absorption and inhalation exposure have been studied.

Skin versus oral absorption rates for the toxic chemicals toluene, ethylbenzene, and styrene were studied in adults and children. These absorption rates appear to be similar to the rates of other chemicals commonly found in our drinking water. The following chart is derived from this research.

Average Skin Absorption vs. Oral Ingestion

	Skin Absorption	Exposure Time	Oral Ingestion	Water Consumed
Adult bathing	63%	15 min.	27%	2 liters
Infant bathing	40%	15 min.	60%	1 liter
Child swimming	88%	1 hour	12%	1 liter
Overall average	64%		36%	

Skin absorption rates are tremendous. People with pools and hot tubs especially take note! These calculations are based on hand skin absorption rates. The hand is a much better barrier against harmful substances, compared with other skin areas which are much more sensitive. This means the true absorption rates are significantly higher.

The above information is reprinted from the book *Healthy Water,* by Martin Fox, Ph.D., published by Healthy Water Research, P. O. Box 173, Portsmouth, NH 03802-0173.

Chlorine is very detrimental to your health. It creates problems in both your blood circulation and your lungs, and as you readily can see from the above research, your body absorbs much more of it from your tub, shower, and pool than you would ever ingest in your drinking water. Therefore, it is imperative for good health that you clean up your household water. The people from Europe will not go into the pools and hot tubs in the United States because they know what the chlorination does to their bodies.

Concerning your municipal tap water, in many cases they cannot get enough chlorine in it to make it safe to ingest, so they also add fluoride and bromines, which just makes more of a toxic soup when you drink it.

So be careful about your water. Some say, "We only have well water out here on our farm, and all of our water has been tested and proven that it's decent to drink." Well, they test the city water and say it's decent to drink, too. The problem is that everybody is downstream from somebody. We're all downstream from the airborne pollution from around the world, and probably every water system in the world got some of the fallout from the Chernobyl accident, simply because it's been up in our atmosphere "falling out" ever since that big nuclear incident in Russia.

You really do need to cleanse your water before you bathe in it. There are some decent filters that you can put on your shower head that will filter out maybe 7,000 or 8,000 gallons before you have to throw it away—these will remove some of the chlorine, but probably not all of it. We have these in our home, and I take one with me whenever I'm traveling. At least I'm able to shower in something that's not totally contaminated with chlorine.

Fluoridation also is dangerous; chlorination is not safe. So, be careful and use a little common sense. If you are using distilled water, make sure you put back the calcium and magnesium that are necessary for the body to function. If you are stripping all the minerals out of your water, consider putting trace minerals and trace elements back into the water before you drink it.

Parasites

There are over 300 different types of parasites. Parasites seem to be dominant in the blood which I examine of just about everyone. You don't see the parasite itself in the blood, but in the blood you see evidence of the parasites that are in their body. The best way to find out if you have parasites it to do a stool examination. It must be sent to a laboratory. The one I am using right now is Smoky Mountain Laboratory (see Appendix C for information about them).

They can tell you if you have tapeworms, hook-worms, pinworms, ringworms, roundworms, or giardia, which is a parasite that lives in nearly all mountain streams and is carried by the beavers. It doesn't bother the beavers, but it gets into all the spring water, and you drink the water and it bothers you! I hear there's pretty much of an epidemic in some of the areas like New York. It's in nearly all the drinking water stages there (as of the writing of this book in 1993).

We've always heard that you don't want to eat uncooked pork because you'll get parasites, but you can get parasites any number of different ways, for example eating raw beef, or barely cooked beef. You can get them from petting your own dog or cat. You actually can get them from walking in the grass from the animal that just dropped them there.

There is one place that people don't realize that they might get parasites, and that's from raw nuts. Now, you may buy raw cashews and think there's nothing wrong with those. Well, just think . . . you didn't shell them, therefore, they were probably shelled by some native in South America or Africa. When he was shelling them, he probably laid them in a pile, because he gets paid so much a pound or sackful for shelling the nuts. The bugs crawl over them and lay their eggs on the raw cashews, and soon they're packaged; and the eggs just lay on them until they get into your body, which is the right temperature and the right moisture content for the eggs to hatch. Then the parasites get into your system and play havoc with your body.

You can get them from raw vegetables if the vegetables are not cleansed properly. And you actually can have parasites transferred during sex. The parasites that live in the colon multiply because they have everything they need—a good food chain, the right temperature—and they can deposit their waste back into your bloodstream and create havoc in your blood. They do affect your immune system, and are present in about 95% of the people whose blood I examine. I don't even have to call it out anymore, I just say there is evidence that makes me suspect that you have parasites in your blood.

I will share with you one very unusual way of getting rid of a tapeworm, if you have no other way of getting rid of it. The way it was carefully described to me—and I knew somebody who had a tapeworm—was that you had to go find some raw milk, neither pasteurized nor homogenized, warm it just a little above body temperature, and put it into a large pan. Then you have to sit in this pan, holding the cheeks of your buttocks open so that the tapeworm will know that the milk is there, and will like the milk better than what it has inside your colon. And you may have to sit there for a half hour for that tapeworm to come out and get into that milk. It's not a very pleasant picture that I'm painting for you. And if you don't wait long enough for the whole tapeworm to come out into the milk, you may break it off. You can break off the head portion, but it will form a new head; also, you have no way of knowing if there is only one tapeworm in there. That's a very colorful way of getting rid of a tapeworm. We had one lady pass a ten-foot tapeworm after that procedure. Believe me, there's got to be a better way!

What I've found in the 703 cleansing (discussed in detail in Chapter 5) is that we're receiving quite a lot of benefit from taking a bacteria called L. Salivarius. This is a friendly bacteria, and in my investigation right now, I'm finding that it is best to take this friendly bacteria every day after the cleanse for at least a month (it wouldn't hurt if you took it forever). Any of the good bacteria that your body needs will multiply and double in number every 20 minutes. But you do not want to go out and eat things like meat that contains antibiotics, or drink chlorinated water, or eat food with preservatives, as all these will kill the good bacteria.

Once you build back this good bacteria, such as L. Salivarius, as God intended it to be in your body, it will actually live in the lining of your colon and your stomach, and it even will migrate into your teeth to help cleanse them. It is hard to believe that a simple little thing like a friendly bacteria can do something this good, but I've found it to be very beneficial.

As you are cleansing your colon, you will wash out the friendly bacteria, along with the harmful things, so they must be replaced. They love oxygen; they are aerobic and they love to live in oxygen. All unfriendly bacteria are anaerobic, which means they can't stand oxygen; oxygen kills them. So just think of it this way: you're putting back some "good guys" after you remove them, and I believe that the good guys, as they multiply, will crowd out the parasites that are in your body, because the parasites will not be able to live there.

I'm seeing evidence of this, and they multiply in great numbers after a few weeks. With ample numbers of friendly bacteria, I believe the body will reject the parasites, because I'm seeing blood actually being cleansed. We are taking nothing directly for the parasites, yet it seems to be working. I'm very encouraged with it. And remember, if you go into a fasting program, the bacteria has an even better chance of doubling every 20 minutes and building a good supply of the "good guys."

Hopefully, you have no parasites; but if you do, you might consider trying this program, because anything else is pretty harsh, and they are pretty tough to get rid of.

Of course, any time you take any antibiotics, you will wipe out your friendly bacteria; any time you drink or bathe in chlorinated water, you'll wipe them out again; and any time you eat processed food that has preservatives in it, you'll wipe them out. It's just like eating stuff you can't digest.

Remember, if the food has preservatives, *nothing* is going to hurt the food, but *everything* is going to hurt your body.

Chapter 3

Firsthand Success Stories

Interview with Julie Hepner

Julie, would you tell us your name and age and something about yourself.

Hi, my name is Julie Hepner and I'm 27 years old. I was diagnosed with metastatic melanoma July, 1990, and since that time, I have had brain surgery and neck surgery, both in July of 1990. Then there wasn't another reoccurrence until September, 1991, when I had an ovary removed, followed in January, 1992 by the removal of a tonsil, and then my small intestine in March of 1992.

You've certainly had a lot of surgery, then, in the last few years.

Yes!

And then we met, around the first of May, 1992.

That's when I first went on the activated oxygen colon cleanse.

And you saw in your blood the things that I showed you. It was pretty dramatic, wasn't it?

Yes, definitely!

And how did that affect you?

It made me definitely want to go on the cleanse and to get the linings [of the colon] out.

Now, have you been to Mexico to one of the clinics?

Yes.

And what did they say?

Well, you know, that I did have cancer and I needed to have some help.

But they wouldn't take you down there, would they?

No.

Because you had too many tumors and too much cancer in your body?

Yes.

And they knew that they couldn't do anything for you because it was too advanced.

That's right.

And you felt like you had tumors and cancers throughout your whole body, right?

Pretty much. It's been all over.

O.K. Of course, right after we met and did your blood study, we told you about the program that I had developed. Then, like a bad guy, I promptly took off to Alaska for three months.

Now, would you tell me some of the things you did while I was gone. I did check on you by phone once in a while, but I honestly didn't believe you were going to do everything that I asked.

Well, right after we met, I went and purchased an ozone generator to add activated oxygen to my water, and I started doing the baths. I think within a week, I had started my first cleanse, and I went on it for the 6½ days. I got rid of a lot of ugly linings during that first cleanse. Then I did juice fasting for a few days after that. I waited a couple of weeks, then I went on the cleanse again. I was on the cleanse off and on throughout the whole time you were away on your trip.

About every three weeks you went back on the cleanse?

Uh-huh.

And you ate primarily fruits and vegetables and drank juices?

Strictly fruits and vegetables and juices.

Now, you did an awful lot of juicing according to the juice book by Gerson, which is great, because I think their juice program is wonderful, and, of course, Norman Walker's and Bernard Jensen's juice programs are about the same. Is there anything particularly special in the juice program that you did? Did you do a certain amount of juice?

Well, I did 13 juices a day, I'm down to 12 a day now. And I've been doing that for a year and two months, so far. I'm basically just juicing fresh vegetables and eating fruits and vegetables.

And, of course, you still clean those fruits and veggies with activated oxygen (ozone) before you ever juice them or eat them, right?

Yes, and I still do the activated oxygen baths.

And you really love the baths?

Yes! It makes you feel really good. Your skin feels really smooth afterward.

And do you feel more energy, just from the baths?

Oh, yes! Definitely.

We had a dentist call us last week complaining that he couldn't sleep because he had waited until 10:30 p.m. to take his bath.

Yes, I can see that happening.

Julie, do you think that this a program for everybody?

For everybody! Whether you have a diseased body or not, everyone should do the cleanse.

And they should do it as often as needed if they have an ache or pain, right?

Yes.

After you went through a total cleansing, we looked at your blood again around September of 1992. We also noticed a difference in your appearance; you actually looked a lot different. You had a sparkle, a glow, it was just totally completely different. But when we reexamined your blood in September, can you remember what I we found?

It was definitely a lot cleaner, the white blood cells were moving a lot faster, my immune system had picked up a lot. Before it was very slow. The whole blood just looked a lot cleaner. All the "spider web-bing" was gone.

And you were pleased?

Yes, very!

Because you had done a lot of hard work in only three months! After that, then you went on some more cleansing in September and October?

Yes, in October.

And when did you go back to your doctor to have your test, about November?

I believe it was November or December of 1992, the same year. And the doctor could not believe his findings. There had been no reoccurrence of the tumors, and the tumors that I did have, he said that they were probably all dead cells.

Now, what kind of testing did he do?

Two MRI's, I've done blood testing, and a CAT scan.

And they all came out negative?

Yes.

And he said that you had only two little tumors that were dead tissue.

Dead tissue, I had them previously, not new ones.

You told me that during the cleansing program, you could feel those were tingling at times and getting real hot, like they were burning. Is that right?

Yes.

And at that point in time, you knew your body was taking care of them?

Yes. . . I think it just takes a little bit longer for the dead tissue to leave the body.

Now, the doctor didn't want to do a biopsy on that dead tumor, because they are very small, about the size of a grape, or smaller?

No, he didn't, although they might be a little bit bigger than that.

A little bit bigger, about the size maybe of an almond or an olive?

Yeah, but they definitely had not gotten any big-ger, and he said they had gotten a little bit smaller, and he believed that they were just dead cells.

Dead cancer cells?

Dead cancer cells.

O.K. Now, have you gone back again since November or December of 1992?

I've had blood tests; I haven't had any more MRI's. I need to go back for an MRI, but in my opinion, I think everything is fine, and I have had the blood testing. I get it done about every two months, and everything is fine with the blood.

Are they primarily doing like a CEA or a . . .

A CBC . . .

Or a CA-125, or something like that, which what they are really testing is how much antigens you have in your body. The more antigens you have, the more cancer that they know the body is fight-ing. Do you know what your readings are?

No, I don't.

Down to one or two, probably?

I think with melanoma it's harder to analyze, that

they can't analyze how much cancer is in the body.

But you have no symptoms, no aches, no pains?

No aches, no pains.

No symptoms whatsoever, no swelling? In fact, you're feeling so good, that you're planning on getting married next year. And what's the date you have picked out for that?

Hopefully, August 20, 1994.

August 20th will be your big celebration, then. How about your boyfriend...does he know all about this?

Oh, yes, he knows all about it, and he truly believes in it, he is very much of a believer.

Now, is he going to go through the cleanse before you get married?

Yes, definitely!

'Cause you're not going to take on a dirty body, right?

Yes, that's right.

Well, Julie, you're an inspiration for a lot of people. I've used your name over and over and told them of your experience, because you are one of the exceptional ones. In fact, if I had to pick someone to have people to follow in cleansing their bodies, it would be you entirely. Is there anything that you can tell people that might help them? Along with your physical cleansing, was there anything else?

I believe in just eating right, to believe in what you're doing, your spiritual...

...you did a total spiritual cleansing, too?

Yes, though probably not as much as you. But just be committed, and have a positive attitude, and believe in what you are doing.

Outstanding!

And, thank you, Bud for everything. I'm glad that we met you and learned about the cleanse.

Well, all praise and glory goes to Jesus, because He brought us together, and it it hadn't been for His Holy Spirit bringing us together, we would never have been able to share what we know. The whole idea now is to share this with the world.

Yes!

We thank you, Julie, and you're an inspiration for all of us, and we certainly do appreciate you.

Thank you, Bud.

By the way, have some of your family gone on this program?

Yes, my dad's gone on the cleanse, my mom's gone on the cleanse, my sister and brother-in-law went on it for a short period of time, and they all benefited from the cleanse.

Any friends, other than family members, who have done this?

I had a friend who went on Jensen's cleanse, and it wasn't as effective because she didn't use the activated oxygen. You definitely need the activated oxygen.

You feel that it's more effective and faster?

Oh, yes, it gets the linings out much faster than without it. I also want to mention that I have a friend, Jackie, who has cancer that has spread all through her body who went on the cleanse. She could tell a dramatic improvement. She also gets regular blood tests, and her cancer rating has gone down, and she does the cleanse about once a month.

She is happy with the progress she is making?

Yes.

But she's not doing it as fast as you did it?

It took her a little longer because the cancer in her body was much stronger than mine, and she was a lot weaker than I was. But she is definitely noticing dramatic improvement. And she's been doing it for almost a year now, as well.

And you think that some cancer patients that are very weak will take a year or so to be totally cleansed?

Yes, it will take longer.

Anything else you want to add, Julie?

Well, again, I'm just really thankful for meeting you and for learning about the cleanse.

You are very welcome, and all praise and glory goes to Jesus, and we do all of this in His name. Amen.

Amen!

Don McAlvany

My name is Don McAlvany. I am in the investment business and have been on Wall Street for the last 25 years and in the political arena for 34 years. I have been writing a financial intelligence newsletter for the last 17 years, and I am a classic

"Triple-A" workaholic-type person.

I am 53 years old this year, and I have spent the last 40 years of my life systematically abusing my body. I cover more ground than most people do. I move very fast; I speak very fast. But over the last five to seven years my body really has begun to run down. I'm a person who knows how to push my adrenal button and run on my adrenals, but even my adrenals have been running out of gas over the last few years.

Over the last 10 to 15 years, people have told me periodically that I looked gray/green. Others have told me that I looked like I was aging very rapidly, and over the last three to five years, I have noticed that for each year that passed, I felt as if I were aging about five years.

It was no surprise when the poor lifestyle, the poor diet, the drinking of large amounts of coffee, getting little sleep, traveling much of the time, and pumping my adrenals overtime all began to catch up with me when I hit my early forties.

Over the last 10 to 15 years, I've tried a number of things to remedy the damage I have done. I got into herbal medicine, and I actually learned a lot of good things from an herbalist in South Africa named Dr. Stanley Dean. He gave me what I certainly would call one of the pieces to the puzzle in the quest for good health.

I began to learn about diet and nutrition, and periodically, I have done good healthy, nutritious-type things . . . interspersed with the bad things I do during my travels, etc., etc. I probably have taken (and this is no joke or exaggeration) from $10,000 to $15,000 worth of various supplements over the last eight to ten years.

But the most frustrating thing is that I have not had a lot of good results from most of the things that I have done. I believe in chiropractic, I believe in kinesiology, I believe in reflexology, I believe in massage, I believe in exercise, I believe in good nutrition, I believe in vitamins, I believe in supplements. . . and I've tried all of the above (more than most people have), and none of it has worked very well. I must admit, until I met Bud Curtis, that I was very, very frustrated about this apparent exercise in futility. Nothing I was doing really was working.

I'm in the investment business; I know how to look at a stock market chart and recognize an uptrend or a downtrend, and for the last five or six years—particularly the last year or two—my body and my sense of well-being definitely have been in a downtrend. So I've been very frustrated. I'll be very honest, in the last six months I've really been praying that God would show me and give me some direction as to what was going wrong with my health. What was the key? Where was the missing link or the missing piece of the puzzle, if you will? Why were all these different pieces that I had been trying to put together just never quite coming together?

Well, in the "fullness of time" in God's great timing, a few months ago He brought Bud Curtis into my life. Bud is a man who lives in California, but we won't hold that against him. He is a man who knows a great deal about the human body, about blood, and about the malfunctioning of blood. But I think his greatest area of expertise is in detoxification of the body. Bud is a dedicated Christian and a man of great concern who would like to go around and really help heal the sick. He feels especially called to minister health to leaders, those who are "out in front," so to speak, trying to help make a difference in our country and in the spiritual realm.

The area on which Bud sheds the most light is the subject of detoxification of our bodies. I have known for some time, as I have done fasting and cleansing, etc. and seen all this dirty gunk on my tongue, that I was very toxic, but I've never really found, either through the fasting or other methods, a successful way to detoxify my body. I have been to probably several dozen alternate medical practitioners. (I gave up on the traditional allopathic medical people years ago.) I have received a little help here and there, but something was wrong . . . the stuff they were giving me just wasn't making much difference!

Well, what I didn't understand—and what Bud since has taught me—is that my body was not absorbing, it was not assimilating, it was not pulling the good stuff out of either my food or the supplements and vitamins I was taking. There was just something wrong. Bud did a blood test on me and showed me a number of alarming things in my body. He showed me the tremendous number of parasites I had, and he showed me the tremendous amount of toxins in my blood. . . and as they say, a picture is worth a thousand words. Pictures don't lie and I saw some things that were most unique and disturbing.

Then he explained to me what was happening in my colon. He told me about the amount of toxification that was there. And even though I've done liver/gallbladder purges, they weren't working because my colon was all "gunked up," and I was just reabsorbing all the poisons that the purges were attempting to dump.

As I began to understand, it was like the lights began to come on, and it became apparent that Bud was supplying the critical missing piece of the puzzle for which I had been searching.

I've been doing a lot of things right; I've been doing a lot of things wrong, but the "lot of things" I was doing right wouldn't quite come together, without the concept of detoxification and the techniques for achieving it.

So, with that information and some gentle and not-so-gentle prompting from Bud and another good friend, Lindsey Williams, several weeks ago I finally did my eight-day detoxification cleanse/ fast.

A most interesting situation! I did activated oxygen water colonics twice a day for eight days. I followed the formula I would say 99.9%, and for a few days during the cleanse I felt pretty badly (I had been advised in advance that I could expect this to occur as I was detoxifying). Indeed, I saw a tremendous amount of dirty grungy things emanate from my body. I would say by the end of the fourth or fifth day, even during the cleanse when you are supposed to feel pretty badly, I began to feel more energy than I had felt in several years.

That had been my number one complaint—not just my bad color, not just the rapid aging, but in fact my number one problem was that I was exhausted all the time. . . I was fatigued and exhausted, virtually all the time. I couldn't play with my kids. I live in the mountains, but I couldn't climb mountains. I tried to ski and I could barely ski. The exhaustion and fatigue that I knew virtually all the time was a really, really frustrating thing.

I noticed during the cleanse that my energy began to come back. If my energy was about a one or a two on a scale of ten, during the cleanse I probably came back to about a four or five. I would say in the weeks that followed the cleanse/detoxification, it went to about a seven, and I will say that I feel better and have more energy than I have had in five to ten years.

We've done some more blood tests; we've examined and analyzed the whole cleanse process that I went through, and we have concluded that I'm not through yet. I probably need to go through at least another eight days, and I probably need to do it two or three times. But I made great progress from the first cleanse —and I would say that I was probably dirtier and more toxic than 98% of the people that Bud would ever encounter. In fact, I have the distinct feeling that I was in the process of dying.

Bud, as well as doctors, have told me that if I didn't make some kind of major changes in my lifestyle, that I could expect to have either a stroke, heart attack, or cancer within the next couple of years. Obviously, that was very discouraging to hear, but also very motivating to try to do something about it.

I feel better at this point than I have felt in the last five to ten years. I am eagerly looking forward to doing the next purge/cleanse/fast in another couple of weeks. And I've seen so much progress, that I'll do it a dozen times if I have to. I'm going to be as clean as a hound's tooth before I get through with this whole thing. I frankly believe when I look in the mirror now, I look normal instead of gray/green. (Friends have told me that my color is better and that I look younger than I have in years.)

I also believe, when I look into that mirror, that I don't look as old as I did before. Now, I'm not saying that this is the fountain of youth, but on the other hand, I believe that this procedure will greatly slow down the aging process, something that my physical abuse to my own body has tremendously accelerated over the last few years. Of course, it would be great if it could roll it back. If Bud can make me look like I'm 39 when I'm 53, we'll just call him the million-dollar man and give him the Nobel Peace Prize or the Nobel Health Prize or something.

I think that Bud Curtis has found the magic key,

the missing link, if you will, the missing piece of the puzzle for a lot of people who really are striving to be healthy and do the right thing, but don't know that as long as their colon is toxic and poisoned, and keeps repoisoning their body, that they simply will not get well.

I think another important aspect of Bud's whole detoxification/cleanse is that he realizes that you must not only cleanse the body physically, but you also must cleanse spiritually. Just as we have economic/financial/ political problems in America, but the root cause of those problems is spiritual, I think probably—I'm beginning to learn this from Bud—the root cause of our physical problem is also spiritual. I think there is a real connection between a spiritual healing and a physical healing, and, of course, in the spiritual sense you also have to clean out the sin and the gunk and the garbage, and the cleansing blood of Jesus Christ does that . . . in His forgiveness after we have accepted Him as our personal Savior. In the physical realm, you have to clean out the scum and the garbage, and that's where detoxification comes in.

I believe that our country is headed into tremendously difficult times, and I believe that we need to strive for medical and physical health self-sufficiency. Alternate medicine and many alternate doctors may be shut down. We may not be able to get supplements. We may not be able to go places where they have great alternate therapies, but if we can learn how to eat, if we can learn how to absorb the right enzymes, if we can learn how to exercise, and most importantly, if we can learn how to detoxify our bodies, then perhaps when real illness does come along, we can use herbal medicines and some other things that it will be very hard for the government to deny us. I believe that it will be possible for us to remain or become medically (or health-wise) self-sufficient. And I think in the days to come that's going to be very, very important.

The first time I met Bud, I really didn't want to meet him. I was scheduled to give a speech in an hour and a half, and I was so tired and exhausted that I just wanted to go back and lie down. But by the providence of God, I did meet with him. He shared this information with me, and we since have become good friends.

I've been into alternate medicine for 15 years, and I believe in it, it's just that it hasn't been working for me (or hasn't been working very well), and I believe that it is now beginning to work. I can say that I'm more "pumped" and more excited about what I'm doing in this whole detoxification process than anything that's come along in a lot of years, and I am very grateful to Bud Curtis, my good friend, for that.

Lindsey Williams

There are two great things that have happened in my life, physically speaking. First, 25 years ago

Lester Roloff introduced me to raw vegetable and fruit juices. The second greatest thing that has happened to my physical body was the day Bud Curtis persuaded me to do a seven-day oxygenated water colonic and fast.

For years I had heard the expression, "Death starts in the colon," and I believed it. But when I saw the rope and the filth that came out of me on the seventh day of an activated oxygen colonic, I became totally convinced that death definitely starts in the colon.

Here is the reason I am so convinced about the necessity of the activated oxygen colonic. For 25 years I have been using enthusiastically a variety of raw vegetable and fruit juices, almost on a daily basis. Twenty-five years ago someone said, "Take carrot, celery, cucumber, beet, pepper, put them all together, and those vegetable juices will do wonders for you." And they did, but 24 to 48 hours after drinking them, my stool always would be red, if the drink contained a sizable amount of beet juice. I asked someone about it at the time, thinking that it was possibly internal bleeding. I said, "Is that normal?" They assured me that it was perfectly normal after you have been drinking beet juice for it to show in your stool 24 to 48 hours later. Right?

Wrong! After cleansing my bowel with the activated oxygen colonics, approximately four months have gone by, and not one time have I ever seen any red in my stool from the beets in my vegetable drinks.

I shall never forget—after the exciting results from my activated oxygen colonic cleansing—I called a friend who, likewise, is very active on raw vegetable and fruit juices, and I told him the story of what had happened. The friend said one word to me: "Absorption." I am fully convinced that a person can take the finest supplements in the world, could even eat the best food available, but if the colon is not able to absorb the nutrients from those supplements or food, then they will not have their intended affect on the body.

The absorption factor is so great, now that I have done the activated oxygen colonics and thoroughly cleansed the colon, that after eating a hearty meal of proper food, I notice immediate energy. I had not noticed that since I was in my twenties. In those days, I could come in tired in the afternoon, eat a meal, and go half the night. By the time I reached my forties, I could eat a hearty meal of good food, and hardly feel any effect. Now, after going through this wonderful cleansing program, I am able to eat a hearty meal, and in a matter of minutes feel the same effect that I did when I was in my teens and twenties.

Now, of course, I am totally convinced that a clean colon is a prerequisite to a healthy body. Bud Curtis' activated oxygen colonic program has done wonders for me. Thanks, Bud!

Chapter 4

Diagnosing Your Problems—Blood and Hair Analysis

Blood Analysis

We examine the blood to determine how healthy or how toxic we are. The Bible tell us in Leviticus 17:14: "...for the life of all flesh is its blood." And remember the story of Cain and Abel...who told the Lord that Cain slew Abel? Now, I know that no one has to tell the Lord anything, but the blood cried out from the ground and told the Lord that Cain had slain Abel.

> ...*The voice of your brother's blood cries out to Me from the ground.*
> Genesis 4:10

I happen to believe that the life energy of the

body is in its blood, and you can see in the blood
the exact condition of your body. Now, the way
I look at blood is far different than the way the
regular medical profession examines it. We are
trying to determine the overall toxicity of your
body, rather than trying to pinpoint any particular
disease, even though there are about 75 different
things you can find from examining a tiny drop
of blood under a dark field microscope. There are
another 75 or so things you can find from doing
a blood crystaline (or dried blood) exam.

Because the blood was so perfectly created,
these things are relatively easy to spot, and if we
kept our bodies clean and toxin-free, our blood
would be clean, and we wouldn't be having these
multitudes of problems that exist today. Keep in
mind the whole premise of this book, as we explained in the beginning, that diseases are not our
problem. . . toxins are our problem. Diseases are
merely symptoms of the root cause, which is
toxemia—a polluted, toxin-saturated body.

When you become toxic in your colon, it will
be reflected immediately in your blood, because
your blood is trying to carry these toxins out of
your system. When your colon is overloaded, the
toxins are deposited in the tissues. Now, when you
clean the colon, that won't automatically clean the
blood, but once the colon is clean and functioning
properly, the blood will begin to cleanse itself,
collecting toxins from the body and dumping them
out through the system which was designed to
expel them, until there are less and less toxins in

the system, followed by cleaner and cleaner blood. During this time, however, it is possible that the blood may appear even dirtier than it did before, because it finally is able to gather up those toxins at the tissue level and rid the body of them, by sending them back out through the liver, colon, etc.

A single red blood cell is about 7 to 8 microns; a white blood cell is about 10 to 30 microns. To give you a point of reference, a micron is 1/25,000 of an inch, so they're pretty small. There are two types of blood examination: live blood and dry blood.

Live-Blood Analysis

Live-blood analysis uses fresh blood under a cover slide, under a dark field condition. You can see activity or indications of parasites present in the system; you also can see a lack of oxygen; you can see protein linkaging and fat particles in the blood. But what we see in nearly everyone's blood is what we call Rouleau. This is a condition discovered by a Dr. Rouleau in Europe, and what you see is that the red blood cells are stacked up like pancakes.

What happens when the blood gets dirty is that the red cells develop this sticky coating. The heart keeps pounding on the blood to get it through the capillaries. The sticky coating is caused by eating foods that the body is not able to digest properly, and it keeps the blood from carrying the right

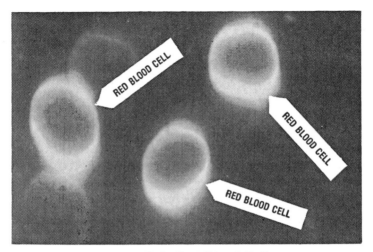

LIVE BLOOD ANALYSIS: Red Blood Cells

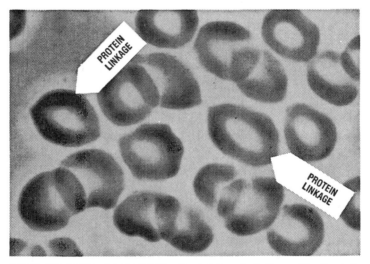

LIVE BLOOD ANALYSIS: Red Blood Cells with Protein Linkage

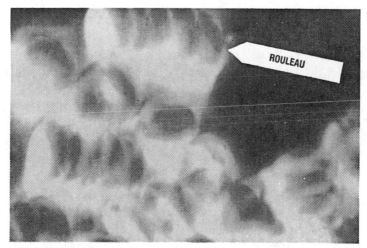

LIVE BLOOD ANALYSIS: Red Blood Cells with Rouleau (nesting)

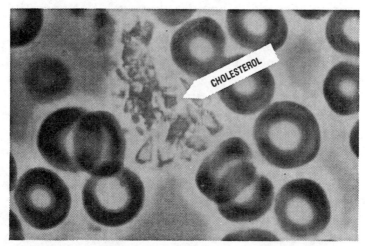

LIVE BLOOD ANALYSIS: Cholesterol among the Red Blood Cells

amount of oxygen and keeps it from having an electrical charge. Red blood cells, when they are really healthy, should be like two magnets. They should come near each other, but never touch. They should be perfectly round, carrying lots of oxygen on the entire surface. When they are sticky they do not carry oxygen; they are stuck together like pancakes, and the only thing showing is the outer edge, which carries very little oxygen.

What we are attempting to do is clean up that blood, so that the red blood cells can begin to carry the oxygen that the body needs at the cellular level for proper metabolism, oxidation, and removal of toxins.

Other things we sometimes see are heavy platelets, heavy cholesterol, and budding candidas or fungal disease. When you have a lot of crenating red blood cells (i.e. dying or shrinking), that can be an indicator that something harmful is going on in the body. But what most people will see in their blood is what we call spicules material. That is when it appears (under the microscope) that there are "spider webs" between and around the red blood cells. This indicates that you have severe bowel and liver toxins. In other words, you have not been eliminating what you should have been eliminating, therefore, you have been building a septic tank within your own body.

In live-blood analysis, we also can see the activity level of the white blood cells. Now, there are many types of white blood cells—there are T-cells, and B-cells, and all types of fancy names—I'm only going to call them white blood cells. Because we can see the activity level of the white blood cells, we have a good indication of the strength of your immune system.

As mentioned above, the red blood cells will give you an indication of parasite activity. Also, the toxins in the blood will destroy the iron that is supposed to be around the red cells to help carry the oxygen. We see a lot of red blood cells with what we call "grease coatings" (hydrogenated oil, grease, butter, fat, etc.) that keep them from doing their job.

We see evidence of chemicals, drugs, pesticides, herbicides, algaecides, all the different types of invaded chemicals that the person is using. Yes, we even can see if you are a "recreational drug" user; I don't think any drug should be considered a "recreation," but that is the common term.

Because I was not happy with a single little dark field microscope, I went into a Zeiss microscope, and then went and studied under Gaston Naessens who developed a condenser. This particular condenser allows you to see more definition, and we are able to see inside a single red blood cell. You actually can see viruses and bacteria forming inside the red blood cell. They invade the red blood cell because it is weak on the outer wall, and they will use that as an incubator to reproduce their own kind...to be released later into your body to create more problems for you. Another large bacteria which you can see is a *motile rod,* and it looks like a series of rods connecting.

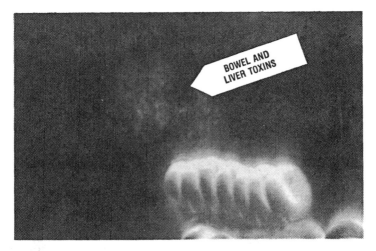

LIVE BLOOD ANALYSIS: Spicules—Bowel and Liver Toxins

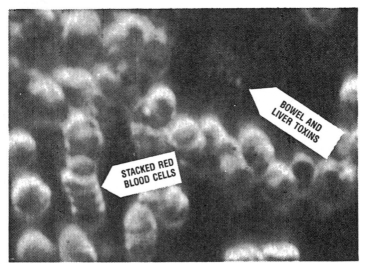

LIVE BLOOD ANALYSIS: Spicules—Bowel and Liver Toxins with stacked Red Blood Cells

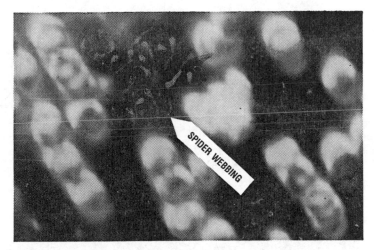

LIVE BLOOD ANALYSIS: With "Spider Webbing"

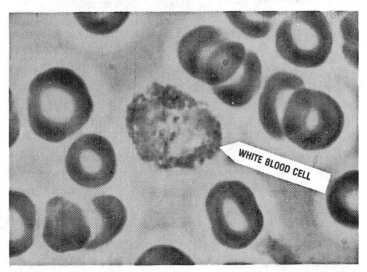

LIVE BLOOD ANALYSIS: White Blood Cell

Although there are hundreds of variations, these are the things you usually find in a live-blood analysis. There is an interesting experiment you can do with a live-blood specimen. Leave it on the microscope in a comfortable temperature for two to three days and watch the growth activity of the bacteria, which sometimes migrate from the red blood cell back out into the blood. Of course, all the red blood cells will die within about an hour, but the parasites, bacteria, and virus forms actually will feed upon the red blood cells and use that as their food chain. You'd be surprised to see how large some of them will grow in just two to three days. It would scare the average person if they didn't know what they were seeing.

Some might say, "The best thing you could do is scare the people, then they would 'shape up.'" People may argue about what they've been eating or what they've been doing to their bodies, but once they see their blood, all arguments stop because they have come face-to-face with irrefutable evidence of their condition. There are other tests, but none as fast or reliable as the blood, because that is an absolutely accurate indicator of the state of your body.

I like to look at it this way. A single red blood cell, while it is alive (and it doesn't live too many days), is a full-time tourist. About every four minutes it travels around the entire system picking up souvenirs. That's why it is an excellent tool to determine the condition of your body.

I'm sure people are curious and would like to

see their blood and find out what types of disease or bacteria are present in it. Well, to me it doesn't really matter because I am of the school that Rife taught, i.e. that all bacteria and viruses are pre-amorphic. Now, that's a big word, but all it really means is that a virus can change to a bacteria and a bacteria to a virus, and they are constantly in a changing form. In much the same way, your body is preamorphic right now; your body is in a state of change—it either is getting healthier or unhealthier. So nothing stays the same. You can watch these bacteria grow and grow. I've never actually seen one change from a virus to a bacteria because a virus is only 1/20 of a micron. Even though Rife possessed the ability in the 1920's and 1930's, the technology has been lost and we are not able to view them today. We do see, however, what we believe are clusters of viruses, even though we have never seen a single virus itself.

In support of the statement that the blood is the life form, we are finding in the blood tiny little somatides, i.e. tiny little electrical energy; they are not bacteria forms, nor virus forms, nor parasite forms—they are only electrical energy. They dance around in your blood, and, in many cases, you can tell exactly how healthy the body is by the quantity of somatides in the blood.

Now, Naessens says that it is the precursor to DNA and RNA; in other words, you have to have those before you can have DNA. He also tells us that it is a cell-reproduction inhibitor, i.e. it tells your cells when to reproduce and when not to.

Something in your body has to tell you when to stop making cells when you don't need anymore, otherwise, you would just continue to grow. These little electrical bursts look like little stars dancing around; they are constantly in motion, and Naessens is convinced that these are the inhibitors. You can take a drop of juice from an orange or any other live food, and you can see the somatides; they are found in everything that is alive.

So, I have to believe that somatides are God-given; it is electrical energy. We actually have cleansed the blood of some people to such a degree that there is very little evidence of somatides in their blood. Now, Naessens teaches that you need a large quantity of somatides in the blood, whereas, I'm of the "old school" that believes that's not quite right. I like Naessens and I believe in his work; he's done a lot of beautiful work and he's been persecuted for it. However, based on my own research, I am of the opinion that somatides are there at the cellular level when you are extremely healthy. When you start destroying the body, e.g. bad food, accumulation of toxins, etc., the somatides come out of the cellular level and into the blood. At that point, yes, you will be able to use the somatides to gauge your health by their number or activity in the blood.

However, when you go back and cleanse the body in detail, the somatides will go back into the cellular level, which is exactly where I think God meant for them to be. I think a few more years of research will determine for sure whether the somatides should be in the blood or at the cellular level.

Dry-Blood Analysis

To perform a dry-blood analysis, a drop of blood is placed on a slide and allowed to dry. If taken properly, a dry-blood analysis can tell you even more about your body than a live-blood analysis.

Unfortunately, the dry-blood analysis is not accepted in the medical community. However, it is very evident by doing the dry-blood analysis that we can tell you very quickly approximately how bad your colon is, if you've been constipated, how much toxins you still have in the body in the colon and reproductive areas. We can tell you just about how loaded your liver is with the toxins you are carrying around in your body. Psychological stress and physical stress can be observed in the dry cell, even if it occurred from four to six months ago (beyond that you don't always see it).

You can see prostrate troubles, lack of Vitamin C, and the inability to assimilate the Vitamin C. However, you actually can change your blood in just a couple of days by taking Vitamin C; take it for a few days and it will show up differently in the blood. You can see a weak thyroid, about where toxins are located in the body and the approximate amount, and about when you can expect to start having physical troubles if you don't get busy cleansing the body right now!

You actually can see a change in the toxic level

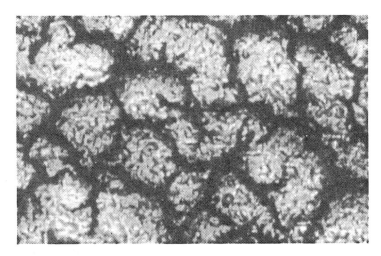

DRY BLOOD ANALYSIS: Sample from good healthy person

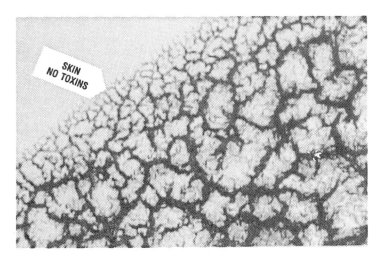

DRY BLOOD ANALYSIS: Skin showing no toxins

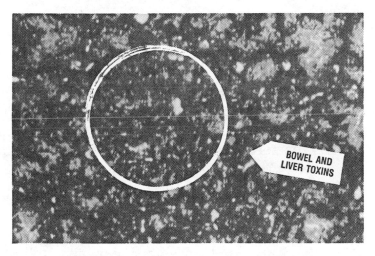

DRY BLOOD ANALYSIS: Showing bowel and liver toxins

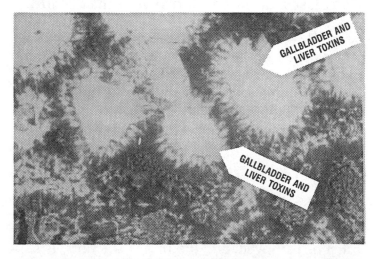

DRY BLOOD ANALYSIS: Showing gallbladder and liver toxins

in a dry-blood analysis taken after only a few days of cleansing. You may see crystals of cholesterol, urine, and other things in the blood—you will see all types of evidence. I know a lot of people would like to spend thousands of dollars going through all the tests to find out every particular bug you have—and I'm going to call them all bugs... viruses, bacteria, parasites, they're all *bugs*. But my attitude is, "Who cares?" because when you cleanse, you rid yourself of all of them, anyway. So don't spend a lot of time and money trying to find out *what* you have—the disease is only a symptom, anyway. The important thing is to be rid of them, so just cleanse your body and all the bugs are gone. It's what we call the shotgun effect. Don't just shoot at one bug or virus, just go in and kill them all. Because if you cleanse the body correctly—clean the blood, clean the colon, clean at the tissue level—the body doesn't need any help to repair. All you have to do is take away the inter-ference...or as we put it in the title of this book, "remove the thorn"...and the body will heal itself.

It's like saying that God didn't make a perfect piece of machinery that would repair itself. Remem-ber, back in Genesis before the Flood people lived from 800 to nearly 1,000 years old. So the body was designed in such a manner that it would re-pair, regenerate, and rebuild itself. Consider some-thing even as delicate as the liver; if half a liver must be removed, and the rest of the body is sup-ported correctly, the liver will reproduce itself and build the liver back. I don't think we should have to go to those extreme conditions. I say, let's give the body a chance and let it repair itself.

We have to stop destroying the body, because it is the temple of God. If you have a dirty temple, then you are not being a very good steward over what God has entrusted to your care, and one day you will have to give account for what you have done to His property, placed under your stewardship.

Hair Analysis

In my opinion, Dr. Eck, Phoenix, Arizona, is the authority on performing hair analysis. Hair analysis, or sampling the hair, is one of the best ways to find out if your body is deficient in vitamins, minerals, elements, and trace minerals, or if it is overloaded on some mineral that shouldn't be there.

It is a very inexpensive process. All you do is take a tablespoon of your hair, near the back of your neck, and submit it for evaluation. The laboratory will send back a detailed analysis of the minerals in your body. Sometimes you have an excess amount of some minerals and metals, rather than a deficiency, and this can be very helpful information.

I believe that hair analysis is a very helpful thing that you can do for yourself—you don't need a doctor to do it. Just follow these simple instructions:

1. Three types of hair will be accepted for analysis.
   a. Head hair cut from the nape of the neck is the primary sample of choice.
   b. Pubic hair can be used as the primary sample only when head hair is not available. Pubic hair also can be used as a cross reference for elevated levels of toxic minerals.
   c. Beard hair may be used only to confirm elevated levels of toxic minerals. Satisfactory comparative values are not available for this sample site. Beard hair cut with an electric razor is not an acceptable sample.

2. Preparation of hair.
   a. Wash the hair using a biodegradable shampoo, rinse thoroughly and dry.
   b. Do not apply hair dressings until after the sample has been cut.
   c. Wait at least four hours before sampling. This allows the hair to reequilibrate following the wash.
   d. Cut the sample before 20 hours.

3. Cutting the hair sample.
   a. Cut small bundles of hair from at least four sites from the nape of the neck.
   b. Trim one inch of hair from the skin end of each bundle until a total of 500 mg. (½ gram) is acquired. This is the sample to be analyzed.

4. Sample rejection.
   a. Sample is less than 200 mg.
   b. Sample obviously contains contaminating media.
   c. Hair appears oily or other dressings have been applied before sampling.
   d. Hair has been permed, colored, or bleached using commercial products. These products permanently damage the existing hair filament. Allow at least 8 weeks for regrowth before sampling.
   e. Hair that has been permed or colored using "home" products is acceptable if the hair has been washed at least 5 times following the treatment. Bleaching always damages the hair filament. Allow 8 weeks for regrowth.
   f. Hair that has been washed with shampoos containing selenium or treated with coloring containing lead acetate are acceptable for analysis. The excessive amounts of selenium and lead are easily discerned during analysis.

The charge for this service is normally $50.00 to $75.00, and they will send you a complete, detailed breakdown of their findings, along with a program of what to eat or not eat, and supplements needed, to get your body better into balance.

Please refer to Appendix B: Available Helps and Where to Locate Them for the information on where to send the sample and other pertinent information.

Chapter 5

How to Become Physically Clean

This book advocates removal of the "thorn" to promote healing, but first we must answer the question, "Just what is the thorn?" In many cases the thorn is sin. If we remove the sin (confess and receive forgiveness), the body will repair itself, as God designed it, or God will heal it. In other cases the thorn is fear. You must replace the fear with faith for God to do His work in your life. If you have prayed many times for your healing, and healing has not come as you think would be good for your body, perhaps God is waiting for you to do something.

It is not likely that God will do for you what He has given you the ability (and instruction in His Word) to do for yourself. Of course, I'm aware that God is sovereign and can intervene miraculously

at any time; in fact, in His mercy, He frequently
does, and one may be totally healed without any
participation on their part other than their faith.
But if that is not the case in your personal circum-
stances, then may I suggest that you consider
taking a "hands-on" approach to the condition of
your health, by consulting and following God's
"Textbook" on nutrition and cleansing and remove the thorn (the things that are harmful to you)
so God can heal. There is much work to be done
for the Lord, and with unhealthy bodies full of
aches, pains, and diseases, we can't give the Lord
our best service.

In order to get your body totally clean, you must
cleanse right down to the cellular level. (Later in
this chapter we will tell you how in great detail.)
Cells are the basic building blocks for the body.
They are designed to regenerate themselves, as
well as burn fuel and give us energy. This process
is called *metabolism,* but this process also produces
a residual waste which must be carried through
our bloodstream to our colon and eliminated.
When the system gets all plugged up, it is the start
of things that are about to go wrong. But let's
address the situation of the cell for a moment.
There are four steps which every cell in the body
should experience daily (or more often). Think of
a box with one function on each side.

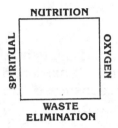

These needs are nutrition, oxygen, waste elimination, and spiritual renewal. If cells do not get what they need, there are devastating results. For example, lack of proper nutrients means lack of "building blocks" for daily cell regeneration. We are oxygen-burning machines. If it doesn't receive enough oxygen, the cell dies and becomes another toxin which must be removed from our tissues. We can survive (poorly) for some time without the other three, but we cannot exist without oxygen. If we don't properly eliminate the waste from our cells, they become polluted and incubators for disease. If we don't feed our mind and body spiritually, we begin to experience negative emotions, which, in turn, bring on detrimental physical effects.

You need at least three sides of the box, or you can expect to go downhill fast!

Mucus and the Colon

There is a widely accepted hypothesis that life and death begin in the colon. A healthy colon is able to absorb nutrients from the blood and eliminate toxins and cellular waste byproducts from the body. However, due to unhealthy eating habits and unhealthy food, over time the colon becomes impacted—much like the inside of a pipe which has been used to pump cement. Like cement, undigested fecal material and wastes from the bloodstream harden, inhibiting proper function of the colon, the interchange of nutrients and toxins from the bloodstream.

When waste products from the blood can't penetrate colon walls that are saturated with hardened feces and mucus linings, they are reabsorbed into the body. This creates a condition known as *auto-intoxification*—literally, the body is poisoning itself. Then the situation is compounded by a myriad of other toxins, originating in our processed foods and our chemical-laden environment.

Symptoms of an unhealthy colon include gas, headaches, irritability, a run-down feeling, chronic fatigue, dulled senses and perceptions, and cold hands and feet, to name only a few. After your immune system has been sufficiently disengaged by all these toxins, then you begin to experience a greater degree of toxemia, namely diseases and organ failure.

Of course, the solution is to cleanse the colon of the years of accumulated debris and mucus linings, then stop putting the toxins into your body to the greatest extent you are able.

Mucus is a normal substance. It is produced in your body to coat the stomach, lubricate the intestines and colon, and aid in elimination. However, the proper foods (fruits and vegetables) eaten raw produce only minimal amounts. On the other hand, eating cooked foods, processed foods, and the wrong foods produces an excessive amount of the mucus. Furthermore, when you eat cooked foods, the body produces mucus, but it is not slippery, it is sticky. So, rather than passing out with the feces, it starts sticking to the colon walls, building up in layers that become hard and rubber-like in consistency. The more harmful things you eat, the more layers you can accumulate.

Of course, these layers prevent the proper exchange of nutrients and toxins, trapping the toxins where they should not stay and preventing the nutrients and oxygen from getting where they need to go for healthy organs and cellular regeneration. Trapped toxins means you will experience toxemia, as well as the diseases that result from it. Instead of clear and slippery, the mucus becomes cloudy, thick, and sticky and will not pass out of the colon. Therefore, the goal of cleansing your body must begin with getting these linings out of your colon.

This is best accomplished by colonic irrigation, also called colemas, with water that has been treated with activated oxygen (ozone), accompanied by a period of fasting and the intake of juices and supplements. In just a few days your system will begin to expel the linings, allowing the proper exchange of nutrients and toxins to resume. These rubber-like "ropes" (sometimes called rubber dams) vary in length and number and can vary in color from green, to gray, to black. Some folks have reported ropes from seven to ten feet long. The average is somewhat shorter. The number of linings can vary from a few to many. (See the photographs; also refer to Dr. Bernard Jensen's book, *Tissue Cleansing Through Bowel Manage-*

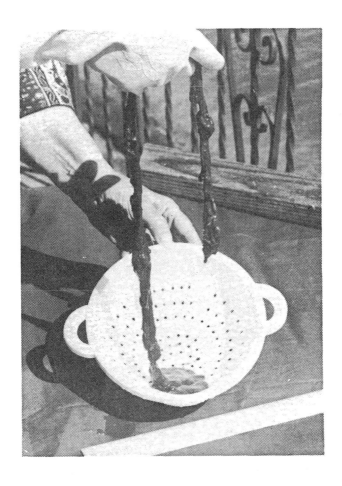

Rubbery linings, frequently referred to as "ropes," eliminated from the colon during the 703 Cleanse Program.

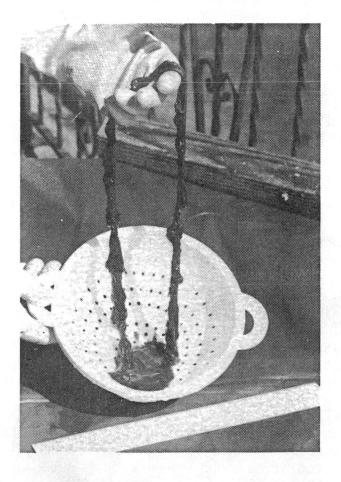

More linings. Several linings of various lengths may be expelled during the seven-day cleansing program using activated oxygen (O₃), which produces the desired results much faster than other methods.

ment, pp. 145-149, for an extensive assortment of these ropes in full color. This book should be available at any good health food store.)

Your polluted blood will begin to appear cleaner as your body goes into a fasting mode, as opposed to its continual digesting mode. However, be advised that as the proper exchange resumes, there will be a period when your blood actually gets "dirtier," as it will reflect the toxins that it now can pick up at the tissue level and dump out of your system. The weaker your body, the less cleansing you can do at one time, but the more you cleanse the cleaner your blood will become and you finally will rid your body of the accumulated toxins. If you are not able to undertake the full regimen (seven days is recommended), then cleanse for a couple of days and give your body a rest period; resume for another couple of days, until you are healthier, then you can go on the seven-day fast and cleanse. After you have detoxified your body, then a maintenance cleanse/fast is recommended about twice a year, with fasting one day a week to give your body an opportunity to rest, get out of the digesting mode, and have a brief cleansing mode.

The Bible recommends fasting, both for health and spiritual purposes, along with prayer and cleansing. Of course, the Bible is our final authority, but comparing contemporary writings can be very enlightening. I'm sure you all are familiar with the Dead Sea Scrolls. The following is a quotation that appears to describe colon cleansing, translated by Edmond Bordeaux Szekely in *The Essene Gospel of Peace.*

> "Seek, therefore, a large trailing gourd,
> having a stalk the length of a man; take out
> its inwards and fill it with water from the river
> which the sun has warmed. Hang it upon the
> branch of a tree, and kneel upon the ground
> before the angel of water, and suffer the end
> of the stalk of the trailing gourd to enter your
> hinder parts, that the water may flow through
> all your bowels . . . . Then let the water run out
> from your body, that it may carry way from
> within it all the unclean and evil-smelling things
> of Satan. And you shall see with your eyes and
> smell with your nose all the abominations and
> uncleannesses which defiled the temple of your
> body; even all the sins which abode in your
> body, tormenting you with all manner of pains
> . . . . Renew your baptizing with water on every
> day of your fast, till the day when you see that
> the water which flows out of you is as pure as
> the river's foam.

Now, it doesn't take an Einstein to figure out
what they are telling us. But let's consider the
effects of living with the linings, in addition to the
obvious things we stated above. There is something we call the hydraulic effect. Have you noticed
how some people always have to go to the bathroom right have they have a big meal? Well, many
people's colons have become so inactive that their
digestive tract is one long tube filled up with food
in various states of digestion, and the only time

they eliminate is when they put some more in and there's no more room for it, so it pushes some out the exit—this is what we call the hydraulic effect.

If we had a clean colon and were eating only those foods that God provided in the Garden of Eden, then we would be passing our food out into the colon area in eight to nine hours, it would stay in the colon area for another three to four hours, then it would be expelled from our body. However, because we do not expel it, it builds up just like layers of an onion, and the body which was designed to be a sewer system becomes a septic tank, and internally we are swimming in our own sewage. That leaves only the lungs, breath, and skin to remove the toxins. That's why some people have extremely bad odors; it's the only way their body has to rid itself of at least a portion of its toxicity.

The best and least expensive way to determine if you have a buildup of linings in your system is to examine your tongue (doctors have been doing it for years!). Don't eat anything after 5:00 p.m., and don't have any meat at that meal. Only drink a small amount of water, and the next morning before you eat, drink, or brush your teeth, go to a mirror and stick out your tongue. If your colon is clogged, you will see a coating on your tongue. How badly it is coated is indicative of how badly your system is operating.

Another simple test is to drink some beet juice. If your stool within the next two days comes out beet red, then most of it did not get absorbed. With a clean and healthy colon, you can drink beet juice without a red stool. This is why some people are overweight—they have to eat far too much food to get any nutrients into their bodies.

It would have been really helpful if God had designed us with a trap door so that we could just reach in and pull out all these linings, but God never intended us to eat the way we do, so now we must deal with the consequences of our disobedience. That is, clean it up or suffer the results . . . the aches, pains, and ultimately disease. Because the mucus that was intended to be eliminated every time we have a bowel movement is building up in the colon, we are having to deal with the results. We are self-destructing in our own septic tank. One of my favorite sayings is, "Either drain the swamp, or fight the aligators!" And these linings are what are preventing you from draining the swamp.

There are several good books out covering the mucus linings in detail. One is by Dr. Christopher: *Dr. Christopher's Cleansing Program.* Another is by Robert Gray: *The Colon Health Handbook.* In addition, there is Dr. Jensen's *Tissue Cleansing Through Bowel Management.* You will find much helpful information in these publications, however, they advocate cleansing through use of herbs and nutrition. . . which will work eventually, but can't begin to compare with the 703 Cleanse for speed and efficacy. Now, I want to acquaint you with some of the foods that I believe are the worst for production of excess mucus. The first is any form of dairy products which produces heavy mucus. Singers are probably most aware of this. . .they are warned early on not to drink milk, eat ice cream, or any other dairy products before they are to sing, as the almost immediate presence of mucus makes it difficult to keep the airways clear enough to sing well. Also wheat, meat of any description, eggs, and citrus fruit produce more mucus than other foods and, therefore, should be eliminated from your diet when you are trying to rid your body of the accumulated mucus linings. Once your colon has been cleansed of the linings, then you can use any of these foods sparingly.

Fasting

Fasting may sound like something the Bible says you are supposed to do. . .well it is. But there are two reasons to fast: physical and spiritual. The Bible advocates both, but in most cases refers to fasting accompanied by prayer. And prayer is helpful in any endeavor, especially physical cleansing. God wants our bodies in good shape, and He is pleased to help us accomplish that goal.

However, the primary reason for fasting for physical results is because the body has two modes: digesting and cleansing/resting. Since we eat perpetually (and usually the wrong things), our bodies seldom get the opportunity to experience the cleansing/resting mode. But fasting is an essential part of the cleansing process, so it is mandatory for the desired results of the 703 Cleanse, which we will describe below.

Healthy Colon

Abnormal Colon

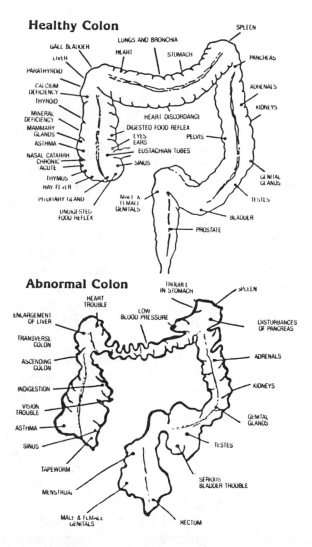

DIAGRAM OF A COLON. While taking a colema, massage your stomach up the left side, then across, then down the right side. You can use a tiny bit of olive oil as a lubricant if desired. This helps the water go all the way to the end of the colon. This diagram also shows the reflex points on the colon for the various organs of the body.

You may be of the opinion that you could never survive a seven-day fast. The Bible speaks of forty-day fasts. Now I don't think any of us wants to go that far, unless God leads us to do so for spiritual reasons, although it might do some of us a lot of good. But anyone can fast a day or two, and most can fast at least a week . . . *we just don't think we can.* You will experience certain physiological effects from fasting. For example, if you fast more than three days, taking only water, your body will start consuming its own flesh; the problem with that is that most of our bodies are so toxic that we would go into an acid mode, and we want to maintain our bodies in an alkaline condition. Therefore, fasting more than three days without juices (fruit and especially vegetable) could be harmful, so we advocate juices and supplements while you are going through the cleansing procedure.

When you are in a cleansing mode, in addition to your colon, you will notice the toxins leaving your body through your breath, urine, and skin. Below we will describe the 703 Colon Cleansing Program and give you a detailed schedule for it, as well as describing the supplements and equipment needed. Also I have included a most helpful report—full of information, tips, suggestions, and observations—by a couple who went through the cleanse (we'll just call them Dr. John and Mary Doe!). In Appendix B we will tell you where all the supplements and equipment may be obtained.

703 Cleansing Program

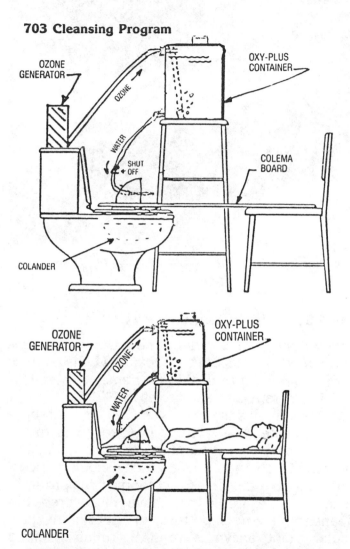

DIAGRAM OF A COLEMA BOARD IN PLACE ON TOILET. You can place a colander in the toilet bowl if you wish to examine the material that comes forth. Use either rubber gloves or a small stick. The end of the board where your head goes should be about one inch higher than the other end. Use a pillow for comfort if desired.

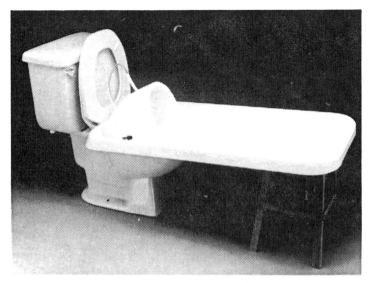

Colema Board (also referred to as a colonic board)

The 703 Colon Cleansing Program

Note: All of the equipment has been described exten-sively in other parts of this book, so in this chapter I will be referring to it only by name.

This program is referred to as the "703" program because you cleanse for seven (7) days with oxy-genated water (O_3). The 703 Cleanse is much faster and more effective than other methods, and the results of ongoing research is being incor-porated into the program as soon as it is properly tested. For example, we have discovered the cleanse works much better with Asperigillus (par-ticular plant enzymes) and Spirulina Pacifica (instead of barley green). The Spirulina Pacific has 96 trace minerals and is the highest-known source of beta carotene.

The cleanse lasts seven days. If you have or

suspect you may have a perforated colon, you should seek competent medical advice before you start this program. During the seven-day cleanse, you take supplements and drink two special drinks about every hour and a half, instead of eating. Because of the enzymes, beet tablets (or crystals), and the drink, you are never hungry, even though your body essentially is in a fasting mode.

In addition, you take two colemas each day. You lie on a special colema board. One end of it rests on a chair or the edge of the bath tub. The other end has a hole in it and is placed on the toilet seat so that it drains down into the toilet.

There is a five-gallon Oxy-Plus Container which has a small tube coming out of it. The tube is inserted through a small hole in the shield part of the colema board. This has an even smaller, disposable tip that is inserted about 2½" to 3" into the anus. This tube remains inserted even when you have to evacuate. It takes a little while (and many evacuations) to empty the Oxy-Plus Container, but you will be amazed at what comes out!

The Oxy-Plus Container is placed about two feet above the board for the first few days and after that a maximum of four feet above the board.

An exciting thing that has been added since Dr. Jensen's book is the use of ozone. Ozone is simply O_3 (now called activated oxygen). There is an extra oxygen atom that will do tremendous work for you when it breaks loose, which it will do. It will kill bacteria, both in the water to be used and in the colon, dissolve carbon, and help to rapidly break loose the multiple layers of linings that are clogging your colon.

As part of the 703 Program, you purchase a small ozone generator. The output hose of this generator is placed into the Oxy-Plus Container. You ozonate the water (let it run) for 15 minutes into the Oxy-Plus Container before you begin your colema. It will totally sterilize the water.

There is also a "clean bath" part of the generator that floats in your tub or spa. Again, you let the generator ozonate the water for 15 minutes before, as well as during your bath. Take a wonderful, relaxing 30-45 minute bath "clean bath" daily, remembering to brush your skin gently but thoroughly several times during the bath. The activated oxygen in the water will aid in removal of dry, dead skin cells and clean the pores so that the skin can aid in the detoxification process. A loofah sponge or mit is an excellent tool for this purpose, as is a natural bristle brush.

After the cleanse is over (seven days, or three days if that is all your body can tolerate), it is recommended that for the first day you only drink fruit and vegetable juices; after that you gradually can add more solid foods. You also will be replacing the friendly bacteria that were washed away with all the bad ones. Be sure to order these and have them on hand before you begin your cleanse.

The benefits of a cleanse are significant. It restores energy, detoxifies the body, lets the liver dump its wastes, the colon now can absorb nutrients and rid toxins, and the body can heal itself. As a result of a colon cleanse, tissue cleansing and blood cleansing occur.

How to Start

First read this book and Dr. Jensen's book. Next, order or buy the supplements and equipment you will need (see Appendix B for locations). Many of these manufacturers will give you a substantial discount if you mention this book and the 703 Cleanse Program. After all of the materials are received and assembled, *set the start date!* Saturday is preferred if you are working. Then start cleansing this vital bowel system.

DOING THE 703 CLEANSE
Information, Tips, Suggestions, and Observations
By Dr. "John and Mary Doe"

'Twas the Night Before Cleansing

We found it was wise to take a 12-cup muffin tin for each of us and fill it with the supplements we would take for the next three days. Since we were going to take supplements four times each day, we oriented the tin with the "three-side" facing us. This gave us three columns of four batches, one column for each day. (Paper cups also work just fine.)

At the time of retiring, we took six S.O.D. tablets. They say that these S.O.D. tablets are a very important part of the cleanse all of the way through, since they put extra oxygen into your bloodstream and help your heart and your liver. We also took two tablets of Sonne's herbal laxative.

The Day Arrives

We took the week off to do the cleanse (but next time we will just keep working). In the four-page report entitled "The 703 Cleansing Program," there are separate schedules for doing the cleanse, working or not.

Upon arising, we took six S.O.D. tablets and dry-brushed our skin all over with a natural bristle brush. This brushing is a vital part of the cleanse. We also brushed our bodies three times during each of the baths . . . but more on the baths later.

Drink No. 2, the apple cider/honey drink, can be taken cold, however, we found that drinking it hot was more delicious and satisfying. We found that heating the water first made it easier to melt the honey off of the spoon and for the honey to dissolve in the water. If you are used to a cup of coffee or tea in the morning, drinking it hot seems to replace that morning cup.

It is a good idea to fix Drink No. 2 *before* you mix Drink No. 1. Drink No. 1 thickens so fast that if you don't drink it immediately, it will get too thick to drink. So after you drink it, follow immediately with Drink No. 2.

Our First Colemas

We filled the five-gallon Oxy-Plus Container with warm water from our shower, using the hose diverter. You can get a portable dishwasher fitting for your faucet and use a regular hose that way. We let the activated oxygen run into the Oxy-Plus Container for 15 minutes before starting the colema. We were concerned about the purity of our water, but were told that the activated oxygen (ozone) running into it for 15 minutes would kill any bacteria in the water.

To help you understand that statement, let us pass on to you what we found out about ozone. Ozone is really O_3. That is, it is a molecule composed of three oxygen atoms (two is the usual number). The third atom is loosely connected to the other two and will break away readily and attack any bacteria or anything with carbon in it. It will oxidize the carbon.

Now to the colema itself. We placed the end of the colon board with the hole in it on the toilet seat and the other end on a chair. (The side of your bathtub could be used, depending on the configuration of your bathroom.) Be sure to have the end on the chair slightly higher than the end on the toilet. We placed a towel on the colon board and placed a comfortable pillow on the chair end.

Then we placed the tube from the Oxy-Plus Container through the hole in the shield of the colon board. *After* it was through the hole, we put the insertion tip into this water tube. (After the colema, we each had a small bottle of 3% hydrogen peroxide [H_2O_2] where we kept our insertion tips between colemas. This sterilized them and acted as a handy place to store them.) We coated the insertion tip with K-Y Jelly® and inserted it. After scooting down toward the toilet as far as we could, it was time to release the first water for our first colema. We found that at the beginning of each colema, we could take very little water before needing to evacuate. (The tip remains inside while you evacuate. It is not necessary to turn the water off—just let it continue to run. The material simply passes around it.) The amount of water we could take began to increase until sometimes we could take so much our stomach would bulge. We found it helpful to massage our stomach while the water was coming in to help the water go up further.

We tried always to leave about 1 " of water in the Oxy-Plus Container to use to wash off the toilet end of the board afterward.

Just so you will be "in the know," while you are on the board and hanging your ten toes over the end of it, some of us call this "surfing." So you can tell others who are "in the know" that you "went surfing today," and they will understand.

We found that the hardest part of the whole process was getting off the board. It is a very awkward process, but gets easier with practice. A friend of ours placed a second chair nearby to help him get off the board.

Examine the Results

Don't expect much the first two days, since primarily you will be getting rid of the food you ate the day or two before you started the cleanse.

After the first two days, we placed a colander in the toilet to catch the solid material. We took an old chopstick and raked through to see what had come out. We were amazed! You could lift up these old linings and sometimes they would be 18 " to 24 " long. Sometimes there were balls about the size of marbles that were made of a black rubbery substance.

Several who have taken the cleanse have passed long rubber-like ropes, some as long as 12 feet. These are made of something the consistency of automobile tire rubber. Next, we dumped the contents of the colander into the toilet and flushed. Placing the empty but dirty colander back into the toilet and flushing again cleaned much of it. The final cleaning was done with a regular toilet brush.

Onward to the Bath

With the ozone machine comes an attachment called the "Clean Bath," which has been nicknamed lovingly "the ozone monster." You see, it has two cute little "eyes" on the top. This floats in your bath water. You will need to disconnect the ozone machine from the tip that goes into the Oxy-Plus Container and attach it to the "monster." You should let the ozone monster run in the full tub 15 to 30 minutes before you get in, and let it continue to run all during the bath.

As you are cleansing (detoxifying), some of the toxins come out through the pores in your skin. These baths are a very important part of the cleanse. The extra oxygen in the bath water both cleans off the toxins and kills the bacteria on your skin, but it also penetrates the skin with pure oxygen. This is why you need to scrub your skin three times during each bath to get rid of the dead skin and bacteria.

Another thing that happens is that your bathtub will get very clean, since the oxygen attacks the scum and film that may have collected and clung to the bottom and sides during the years. We have a large inlaid tile tub and had trouble with stains and scum from our hard water. The first time we put the monster into the tub, there was actually a coating of silt on the bottom of the tub! We were concerned that perhaps our water filters had gone bad. The next time there was less silt. Soon it was all gone and the bottom and sides of the tub were sparkling clean, as was the water!

The bath each day was one thing that we really looked forward to. We felt energized and refreshed after each one. Our bodies felt so clean and nice, that we are sure you will enjoy the baths, too. By the way, you don't necessarily want to feel this envigorated when you want to sleep, so it is advisable *not* to take them too close to bedtime. Some people who have done so have reported that they have trouble getting to sleep.

If you undertake this program while you are trying to work, probably you will be able to do only one bath a day. That is all right, but do not let anything keep you from that one fabulous bath. We were able to take only one bath a day, although two would have been ideal.

Taking the Supplements

We already have discussed the two drinks that you drink fives times each day. These are a very important part of the cleanse. The apple juice, honey, and apple cider vinegar help keep you from getting hungry and provide needed nutrients for your body, as well as helping you detoxify. We never got hungry during the entire seven days of the cleanse, even though it is considered a seven-day fast.

Likewise, taking the supplements is a necessary part of the cleanse. The Vitamin C., Spirulina Pacifica, and the multivitamin also provide needed nutrition and help keep you from getting hungry. The Bio-Energy 321 and 649 provide enzymes that help you digest undigested proteins, and they help the colon to release the mucus linings.

The program calls for beet tablets or crystals. We dissolved a tablespoon of beet crystals in water and used that as the liquid with which we took the rest of our supplements. It makes a nice drink.

Put the Calphonite in your morning and evening drinks (either Drink No. 1 or No. 2).

A word about niacin is in order. After taking it, many people get some degree of "niacin flush," with some of their skin turning red and tingling. Mary got such a flush that she had to cut her niacin intake in half. But if niacin is causing your skin to flush, they say that it is because of improved circulation throughout the body and to the colon, which is helpful to the cleanse.

Take More S.O.D.

We were told that if you get a little woozy or you are feeling just plain poorly during the cleanse, take some extra S.O.D. tablets. These are wonderful little helpers and are something that you might want to consider taking regularly after the cleanse is over. Check with your nutritional advisor to see if it fits with your regular supplements.

The S.O.D. is an anti-oxidant which stops cell deterioration, helps get oxygen to the cellular level, and helps your body handle the effects of the dramatically increased detoxification that is happening in your body. If you are experiencing an energy slump, it helps to take some additional S.O.D.

Coming Off the Cleanse

Your body has just had seven wonderful days of cleansing and has taken in no solid food. It is unwise to jump right back in and start eating your regular solid-food meals right away. It is recommended that for the first day after the cleanse that you restrict your diet to vegetable and fruit juices.

The second day after the cleanse, begin to add in some steamed vegetables and salads. By day three, you can begin to ease back into solid food.

During the cleanse, many of the friendly bacteria (flora) got flushed out of your colon, along with the bad stuff. It is very important for two weeks following the cleanse to take one or two capsules of D.D.S. No. 1 Lactobacillus Acidophilus three times each day. You also need to take four capsules of L. Salivarius twice each day. These will help replenish the flora (good bacteria) in your colon.

We did not realize that we needed these until the fifth day of the cleanse, so we had to have them rush-shipped to us. This was an unnecessary expense. So be sure to order these at the same time you order your supplements for the cleanse.

Repeating the Cleanse

The question often arises as to whether the cleanse should be repeated and, if so, how many times and how often. You should let your body rest for six to eight weeks before repeating the cleanse. One reason is that the detoxifying process will continue in your body after the cleanse is over.

Much of the contaminants in your blood can now be dumped by the liver into the colon. Whereas before, if your colon was very clogged, the liver tried to dump the wastes there, but couldn't. Some of the sewage was absorbed back into the body and some of it wound up back in the bloodstream. Give the body time to do its own cleaning before starting on another cleanse.

As to how many cleanses are required to cleanse your colon properly, that will vary with the individual, depends on how badly the colon is lined, and many other personal considerations. We understand that for most people in a western country it will take at least two or three cleanses to get rid of the majority of the undesirables. For some, it may take as many as five or six. You will have to be the judge of that. One criteria to use is cleanse until the horrible bad-looking stuff no longer comes out.

Once you are cleansed to your satisfaction, then repeating one cleanse each year should be adequate to keep your colon clean.

For Believers in Jesus Christ

If you are a follower of Jesus Christ, praying while surfing seems to accelerate the process of cleansing, according to many Christians who have done a cleanse. You also can put on one of your favorite music tapes while surfing. It can be a spiritually renewing experience, as well as a physically renewing time.

Our Evaluation and Recommendation

We had our blood tested where we could see on a television monitor our red and white blood cells. John's red cells were stacked up like pancakes, there was much "spider webbing" (a residue indicating the probable presence of colon and liver toxins) between the red blood cells, and his white cells (responsible for the immune responses) were very inactive, not moving at all and "boiling" only on about 25% of the surface. After the cleanse, we had our blood retested. Most of the pancaking was gone and the cells were nice and round. Much of the "spider webs" were gone, and his white cells were amazing. They were moving all around like snails, boiling all over with productive activity and eating all of the trash in sight, just as they should be doing. The cleanse made quite a difference and significantly improved John's immune system.

Mary's dry blood test before the cleanse had many "lakes," indicating toxic accumulations. After the cleanse, almost all of the "lakes" were gone, showing that much detoxification had occurred. While massaging her stomach during the colemas, Mary found three very hard spots on the colon that were sore. After six days of the cleanse (and passing some significant linings and other undesirable matter) two of these spots were gone and no longer tender.

Each of us lost about eight pounds during the cleanse. Basically, this has stayed off because we were getting rid of compacted waste that we had been carrying around for years.

We both felt an increase in energy, even exhilaration at times. We no longer experienced our usual afternoon sag.

We would highly recommend a 703 Cleanse. It is not a "cure-all" and no medical claims are made for it. However, we have found that it has helped our overall health, and we are looking forward to our second cleanse.

It was a good experience for us, doing it together. We both had someone to encourage us and to share the experience. It was fun making the drinks together. John made the honey/vinegar drink, while Mary got the mixings for Drink No. 1 ready, adding the Sonne's No. 9 powder into the blender or shake container when John had completed making Drink No. 2. We hope that the cleanse will be as good an experience for you. Our prayer for you is . . .

> May God make you clean both physically and spiritually. May He give you peace through the Prince of Peace, His Son, Jesus!

703 Cleansing Schedules

NOTE: It is important to remember to close the ileocecal valve before beginning your colema (this is the valve separating the small intestine from the colon). If this procedure is omitted, it can produce most unpleasant results when material is allowed to flow from the colon into the small intestine (you could be very ill for a day or two). To perform this procedure, place your right hand (with fingers extended) between and above the breast and raise your right elbow, turning hand in clockwise motion (looking at the body).

Cleanse Schedule

The night before the cleanse, take two cascara sagrada tablets (a laxative available at any drug store).

6:30	6 S.O.D.
7:00	Drinks No. 1 and No. 2
7:45	Start ozone into five-gallon Oxy-Plus Container
8:00	Start colema
8:30	Take supplements

10:00	Drinks No. 1 and No. 2
11:30	Take supplements
1:00	Drinks No. 1 and No. 2
2:30	Take supplements
3:00	Optional *broth or tea
4:00	Drinks No. 1 and No. 2
5:30	Take supplements
5:45	Start ozone into five-gallon Oxy-Plus Container
6:00	Start colema
7:00	Drinks No. 1 and No. 2

*Hidden Valley Seasoning Broth
(1 Tbsp. in a cup of hot water)

Assistance is Available

If you have any questions about the 703 program, you may contact Pat Lee or Linda Getty. Pat has helped hundreds of people through the program and Linda assists different groups weekly at different locations to go through the program. They also can make available to you the different equipment and supplies you will need. Refer to Appendix B: Available Helps and Where to Locate Them for complete information.

Cleanse Supplements

It is helpful to understand why you are taking these supplements—their purpose and how they function —therefore, a brief explanation of each is furnished below.

Cascara Sagrada: a natural laxative taken the night before the cleanse to disperse any remaining food particles in the intestinal tract before you begin your activated oxygen colema.

S.O.D. (Bio-Guard): Superoxide Dismutase is an anti-oxidant which helps in removing toxins from the body and stops cell deterioration.

Apple juice: very good for the bowel because it is high in pectin, which is a moisture-holding substance.

Apple cider vinegar: very high in potassium and good to relieve any mucus or catarrhal conditions. Helps provide needed nutrients to muscle tissue.

Beet tablets or crystals: a slight laxative that works well with the liver, promoting the cleansing of that organ.

Niacin: produces hot, red flush and is used to push the blood deep into underactive tissues so that they can be strengthened with vital nutrients.

Minerals: formula stimulates new cell growth.

Spirulina Pacifica: bluegreen algae is highest source of beta-carotene, plus 96 trace minerals that help in the cleansing process.

Calphonite: a colloidal calcium.

Dulse: quickens the thyroid gland and speeds up the metabolism, while bringing heat to the body causing the blood to circulate deeper.

Sonne's No. 7 (Bentonite): a clay suspended in

water. It is very useful in absorbing toxic substances. It can absorb 40 times it own weight
in toxic substances. It acts like a sponge, mop-
ping up undesirable debris. It has a great effect
on the mucus membrane, loosening it and
releasing it faster.

Sonne's No. 9 (Intestinal Cleanser): this material
holds moisture well and attaches itself to the
mucus lining, making it soft and loose so it will
move away from the bowel wall.

Flax seed oil: contains essential fatty acids (EFA)
which boost metabolism, metabolic rate, energy
production, and oxygen uptake, among other
benefits.

Enzymes (Aspergillus—plant enzymes): help in the
digestion of the supplements and undigested
food in blood and cells of body.

L. Salivarius: taken after the seven-day cleanse;
doubles its population of flora (friendly bacteria)
in the small intestine every 20 minutes.

Acidophilus: taken after the seven-day cleanse;
used to reestablish the flora in the colon.

Hidden Valley Seasoning Broth: optional broth drink
to ease hunger symptoms during the fast.
1 Tbsp. in 1 cup hot water.

SUPPLEMENT	QUANTITY / POTENCY

30 Minutes Before Early Morning Supplements

S.O.D. - A o+   6

Early Morning

Vitamin C	1/1000 mg
Niacin	1/100 mg (1st day); 2/100 mg after
Bio-Energy 321	2
(or Similase)	
Spirulina Pacifica	9 6
Multivitamin	1
Bio-Energy 649	3
(or M6)	
Calphonite	2 Tbsp. in A.M. drink
Beet crystals	1 Tbsp. in 10 oz. water
Dulse	2 tablets or 1 dropper

Late Morning & Afternoon (coffee breaks)

Vitamin C	1/1000 mg
Niacin	1/100 mg (1st day); 2/100 mg after
Bio-Energy 321	2
(or Similase)	
Spirulina Pacifica	9 6
Multivitamin	1
Bio-Energy 649	3
(or M6)	
Beet crystals	1 Tbsp. in 10 oz. water
Dulse	2 tablets or 1 dropper

Evening (as soon as you arrive at home)

Vitamin C	1/1000 mg
Niacin	1/100 mg (1st day); 2/100 mg after
Bio-Energy 321	2
(or Similase)	

Spirulina Pacifica 2 b
Multivitamin   1
Bio-Energy 649   3
   (or M6)
Calphonite   2 Tbsp. in P.M. drink
Flax seed oil   5 capsules
Beet crystals   1 Tbsp. in 10 oz. water
Dulse   2 tablets or 1 dropper

Drink Recipes

The drinks are taken in sequence, with Drink No. 2 following immediately after Drink No. 1. However, because Drink No. 1 thickens almost immediately, it is wise to prepare Drink No. 2 first, so it is ready to go as soon as you have swallowed Drink No. 1.

Drink No. 1

Put 10 oz. water in blender
Add 4 oz. apple juice
Add 2 Tbsp. of Sonne's #7
Add 1 Tbsp. of Sonne's #9
Mix and drink immediately
because it will thicken too
much if you don't

Drink No. 2

Put 10 oz. water in a mug
Heat in microwave for
   1½ min.
Add 1 Tbsp. apple cider
   vinegar
Add 1 Tbsp. honey
   (raw, unfiltered)

After the Cleanse is Over

Drink juices for the first day and gradually ease into solid food.

3 times daily — 2 caps D.D.S. #1 Lactobacillus Acidophilus
3 times daily — 4 caps of L. Salivarius for the first week.

3 times daily — 2 caps of L. Salivarius for the second week. Thereafter, 2 caps of L. Salivarius a day until you use the remainder of the bottle.

Nervous Stomach

Everyone is susceptible, however, women are more prone to this than men. I find that more than 50% of women have what I consider a very nervous stomach. They worry, and when they do worry they tie up their stomachs in knots. There is a very simple little exercise they can use to relax their stomachs. Sometimes even when they are asleep their stomachs won't relax. Here's what you do. Lie on your back and locate a spot on your abdomen approximately 1 " above and 1 " to the left of your belly button. Take one of your fingers and push straight in very hard at that point. When you do, you will find a very sore spot there, almost like something is inflamed. That's the place to which people are referring when they say something hit them in the pit of their stomachs. When that spot is tied up in knots from worry or stress, no digestion takes place, no matter what you are taking or what you are doing.

This procedure must be done the last thing before you go to sleep. If you can't sleep and get up and wander around, you must repeat the procedure, or if you lie in bed and worry for two hours without going to sleep, you should repeat the procedure. If you just get up in the middle of the night to go potty, then go straight back to sleep, it is not necessary to repeat the process.

Locate the tender spot and push on it for a mini-mum of three minutes (which will seem like an eternity when you are pushing in on a painful area), then release it, turn over, and go to sleep. Do this for at least three nights; I recommend you do it for two to three weeks. By that time things will be flowing normally in there. It will feel like the water flowing through a garden hose when you hold it between your fingers, but it will free up the "knot" so that proper digestion can go on during the night, leaving you ready to begin the next day ready to eat again.

God is just—I pay only for my physical sins... by aches, pains, and disease. You pay for yours and I pay for mine. Someday we will stand before the throne of God to be judged for our spiritual condition, according to our relationship with His Son, Jesus Christ, and the things we've said and done—but I believe that we are judged daily by our aches and pains for what we do to the body which He placed in our care.

Chapter 6

How to Become Spiritually Clean

Spiritual cleansing must be based upon a firm foundation; therefore, the very first thing you must do to become spiritually clean is to *accept that the Bible is the inspired Word of God.*

Second, you must *accept Jesus as your personal Lord and Savior,* trusting that through His blood you are saved. If you wholeheartedly repent of your sins (repent does not mean to "be sorry for," although it is likely that you will be sorry when you recognize your sinful condition; repent means turn and go in the opposite direction), ask for forgiveness, and open your heart to Jesus, He will come in. You will become what is referred to as a "born-again Christian." And even though the world may ridicule that term, it is a good thing,

not a bad one, because Jesus said unless a man
be born again he cannot enter into the kingdom
of God. So you have now become adopted into
the family of God and are an heir who will inherit
a place in that kingdom someday. Jesus told His
followers before His ascension into heaven that "I
am going to prepare a place for you, that where
I am, there you may be also. And if I go, I will come
again and receive you unto Myself."

After a relationship has been established, in
order for it to grow and mature there must be communication. Communication between God and the
Christian is called *prayer*. The Bible tells us to
"pray without ceasing." As we learned above, if we
open our heart, Jesus will come in. . . His Holy
Spirit lives right inside us. The Bible in many
places calls our body the *temple* of God. So with
the Holy Spirit right inside us, prayer is just a heart-
beat away at all times. Jesus said He was sending
the Holy Spirit to be our comforter (in Greek that
is *parakletos,* one who is along side). So talk with
God many times throughout the day, just as if God
were right there along side of you at all times,
because He is! Converse with Him, get to know
Him, but don't do all the talking. Remember, con-
versation is a two-way street, you must learn to
listen, as well as talk.

When you become a Christian, you begin to live
in the "real" world, not the world of the five senses,
which is only the temporal world. This means that

your life now is to be led by the Spirit, rather than your senses. In your own strength, this is not possible, but if you ask the Lord to nail your fleshly appetites and human will to His cross each day, you will begin to experience the joy of walking in the Spirit. With the assistance of the Holy Spirit, you will be able to recognize and resist the works of the devil as he tries to tear down your faith.

God wants to hear from us. He delights in our love for Him, and He tells us to enter boldly into His presence, making our needs and petitions known to Him. However, that doesn't mean we just are to become "Gimme" Christians. The Word of God tells us how to approach Him. First, we are to "enter into His gates with thanksgiving and into His courts with praise." So express your love and gratitude to the Lord for Who He is, because He is worthy of our praise, as well as with thankfulness for all He has done for us. . . even for the routine things which we usually take for granted. Communication is essential for building a strong relationship, so don't neglect frequent, sincere prayer.

Next, we need to see what God has to say to us in His written Word, the Bible. All the instructions for successful godly living are in there. So read the Bible in two ways. First, read it devotionally, that is, just read and meditate on it, and let the Holy Spirit within you illumine the things He has for you in the Word that day for your spiritual growth and enlightenment, the *Rhema* Word. Next, read the Bible like a textbook—study it carefully for instructions in how to live your daily life, how to conduct your business, raise your family, or care for your body.

When God gives us instruction in how to do something, we should be obedient, not rebellious, as He created us and He alone knows what is best for us. God's Word gives us instruction in how to become clean both physically and spiritually, and this chapter deals with spiritual cleansing; however, if God's Word instructs you to become clean physically (see Chapter Five) and you refuse to obey, then that disobedience has an affect on you spiritually, as well as physically.

Another thing we are instructed to do is commit the Word to memory, so that we will know what it says when we don't have a copy handy, but even more important, so that it will become engrained in your spirit, actually become a part of you. "Thy Word have I hid in my heart that I might not sin against Thee." "Thy Word is a lamp unto my feet and a light unto my pathway." The goal of a Christian is to become more Christ-like as you grow in your Christian life, and without the Word buried deeply in your spirit, that will be next to impossible.

Now, I realize that most of us consider our brain to be a sieve, with what we put in there leaking out almost as fast as we put it in. . .and with most information, that may be true. But in the Bible we have a promise from God that the Holy Spirit will "bring to our remembrance" those things that we need at the time we need them. However, if we don't ever study the Word and put into our memory banks what it teaches us, then when we need the

Holy Spirit to call something useful to our remembrance, the request may come back stamped "NSF—Insufficient Funds."

Once we have become a Christian, God will let the Holy Spirit convict us whenever we disobey or sin in some way—in other words, your conscience will start to bother you "big time." Be quick to respond to His prompting and confess at once and receive forgiveness. The Holy Spirit begins "cleaning house" in our lives from the day we first accept Jesus as our Savior. He will nudge you gently and make you feel uncomfortable with your old way of life, so that you will find much more joy in your new way of life. When His work is done, you will be a *clean temple.* In the beginning, as a little child who is learning to walk, you will fall down from time to time (stumble back into your old ways), but don't stay down. Get up and keep trying till you can run in the race.

As you repent promptly each time, your failures will become further and further apart. That doesn't mean you will achieve perfection, although we are admonished to strive for it; there will be different areas in your life on which the Holy Spirit will work, striving to make us ever more Christ-like.

But regular spiritual cleansing is necessary and exceedingly simple. God's Word says, "If we confess our sins, He is faithful and just to forgive us our sins, and to cleanse us from all unrighteousness" (I John 1:9). Also, "If anyone sins, we have an Advocate with the Father, Jesus Christ the righteous" (I John 2:1). An advocate is an attorney;

in other words, Jesus is at the right hand of God making intercession for us...being our attorney. And God has promised to remove our sins as far as the east is from the west and *remember them no more*. Once they are under Christ's blood, they are forgotten...blotted out of our account in God's books.

There is one thing to remember about forgiven sins: even though God forgets them, we may have trouble doing so. And just as we have an Advocate in Jesus Christ, we also have an adversary in the devil, Satan, who is called "the accuser of the brethren." It is his purpose to accuse us before God of everything unconfessed and unforgiven in our lives. But once it is confessed, forgiven, and *forgotten* by God, then Satan's only other recourse is to hassle us about our past sins, since we lack the mental ability to *choose* to forget things—in fact, it usually works out that the harder we try to forget something, the more we remember it. He can't lay those sins back on us, but if he burdens us down with guilt, then he can make us to become ineffective in our Christian lives and poor witnesses of the redemptive power of Christ.

There is a saying that has been used so often in Christian circles that it almost has become a cliche...but it is true, nonetheless. There is a difference between conviction and condemnation. Conviction is from the Holy Spirit about sin in our life, urging us to confess and be forgiven, and keep our temple clean. Condemnation, on the other hand, is from the devil, trying to lay a guilt-trip on us, telling us we're not forgiven, and we're just kidding ourselves. He wants us to roll over and play dead; since he has lost our souls, he will settle for keeping us miserable, useless Christians all our lives. We must remember (there's that word again . . . you have to put the knowledge in your memory bank if you are going to be able to make a "withdrawal" when you need it!) that the Word says that Satan is a liar and the father of lies. In other words, you can't believe a thing he says. Another thing to "remember" is that Jesus gave the believer authority over the devil and his armies, so when you have confessed your sin and received forgiveness (and therefore, what you feel must be *condemnation*), rebuke Satan in the name of Jesus and tell him to get behind you. One more thing to "remember" is that the Word promises us that if we resist the devil, he must flee from us.

My spirit is saved through Jesus; my mind is being saved through Jesus; my body will be saved through Jesus. It takes very little knowledge to do what He commands. Remember, He only gives us a few simple rules. And the Ten Commandments can be summed up in the following: forgive all of the people who offend you, not when you want to, but as it happens daily; accept Him; love everyone, even those who try to do you harm.

It is through the blood of Jesus, the Spotless Lamb sacrificed for our sins, and by His grace that we can be saved. The Lord only needs people who are willing to follow His commandments out of *love* for Him, not from duty or because He requires it. Repent, ask for forgiveness, believe in Him, renew your soul daily through study of the Word, and share His salvation with other people. Do not be ashamed of becoming a Christian; acknowledge who you are through Jesus. Jesus said if we confess Him before men, He would confess us before the Father.

This has been a brief study in spiritual cleansing, but there is enough information here for an unbeliever to understand the plan of salvation and invite Jesus to become his Savior. That's where true spiritual cleansing begins. If you are just now at this stage in your spiritual cleansing, let me urge you to take that first step, then seek out a group of other believers where you can fellowship and worship, where the uncompromised Word of God is taught, and where you can grow into a mature Christian...sharing your newfound faith with others who need to learn of the Lord.

And above all else, keep that "temple" clean! ...physically, of course, but especially spiritually.

Chapter 7

The Importance of Enzymes

Most people who have been eating cooked foods and have not been on a raw food diet are bankrupt in enzymes.

To me, enzymes are a God-given element that your body has to have to properly digest and assimilate nutrients from the food you eat—in other words, to keep you healthy. In raw food you get enzymes, just as you get vitamins and minerals. But if your food is cooked, your body has to give up the vitamins, minerals, and enzymes and just get that food processed through your body.

A lot of people consider enzymes as nothing less than the actual substance that makes life possible. The reason we need enzymes is because the bio-chemical reaction in the body will not function without them. Every organ in our bodies, all the tissues and cells, are run on a metabolic process. The "driver" of this metabolic process is metabolic enzymes. In order for you to be able to handle the food that you eat—the proteins, carbohydrates, and fats—your body needs enzymes to process them. If you do not have sufficient enzymes available, your body cannot process properly what you ingest, and it will end up in your bloodstream, creating havoc in your body.

The biochemical reaction that takes place will allow the enzymes to work only at a certain pH and a certain temperature, as food enters your digestive tract. And when it's not in the right pH and temperature range, the enzymes are deactivated. However, when enzymes are present, and the temperature and pH are correct in your digestive tract, the enzymes go to work (the metabolic process). But any time you heat food above 104°F to 120°F, you have killed all the enzymes. They cannot exist above 120°F. All the microwaving and all the heavy cooking is like pasteurizing your food. When you do that, you've allowed all the "good guys" in your food to be destroyed, and your body has to give deplete its enzyme reserves to process your food intake. What you have done is "bankrupt" your deposit of enzymes.

There are over 5,000 different enzymes. Some of them have been identified, but it seems we only talk about a few of them. The one about which you will hear the most is one that digests protein. It is called *protease*. That one is the most frequently absent in the people whose blood we test, because in the test we find undigested protein linkaging around the red blood cells. This means that they are eating a protein that their body cannot digest, or they are eating too much of the wrong type of protein, and it has coated the red blood cells. Therefore, in order to help them get that out of their systems, we encourage them to take an enzyme that will help digest that protein.

The fat molecules that we also see in the blood must have the *lipase* enzyme present in order to digest the fat. Well, the Bible tells you not to eat the fat of the animals, but if you are eating it anyway, you must have a large amount of lipase.

The other enzyme about which you may hear a lot is called *amylase,* and it is required for the digestion of carbohydrates. Amylase is very important because nearly everything you eat will end up turning into carbohydrates, or blood sugar. I think we eat entirely too much of the simple carbohydrates, those things that have been demineralized and devitaminized, so you will need a lot more amylase enzymes if you do eat those types (which means the white flours, white sugar, etc.).

Cellulase is the enzyme that digests the fiber. There are about 22 different digestive enzymes that are produced by the pancreas. A lot of people think, "I don't need to take enzymes because my body is going to produce all the enzymes I need." Wrong! If you are eating perfectly, just like the Garden of Eden (Gen. 1:29), that is true. But that means ever since "Day one" (about nine months before you were actually born, since you get mother's nutrients before that) you have been eating only the food that's good for you, only food that has not been polluted with the things from our environment—directly or indirectly—grown in nontoxic ground, and eaten raw. In the unlikely event that you could be that person, then, yes, your body will produce all the enzymes you need.

But because of the things we do to our bodies and the environment in which we live, I don't know of anybody who doesn't need to supplement their enzymes, especially if you are going to have a particular meal that is not 100% raw food nor 100% nutritional food. You certainly should be taking enzymes with the meal to help digest the food, because your body will be unable to digest it without assistance.

Some people take *pancreatin,* which is an animal enzyme. I find nothing wrong with this, but again, I believe that the good enzymes come from plant food, rather than animals. You will notice in the wild animal kingdom, for example when a lion kills another animal, the first thing he does is break open the belly and eat all the organs. The reason is that he is after the enzymes, vitamins, and minerals that are heaviest in the organ areas. Lions were created with the instincts to know that the best nutrients are not in the flesh parts, they are in the organs.

Now, that doesn't sound very appetizing to me. What we are really searching for is a way to help the body, so it can do a better job of handling the food that you are ingesting. The whole ball game boils down to trying to build a perfect condition in our body where every cell and every organ is working together in harmony—this is called *homeostasis,* which means it is like a fine orchestra. All the instruments are playing together and making beautiful music.

As we continue to do bad things to our bodies, pretty soon the only thing left playing is the bass drum. Now, the bass drum doesn't make beautiful music, like the full orchestra. So, the best homeostasis is when everything that *God made* for your body is *working in harmony* in your body *for the benefit* of your body, so that you can become very healthy. Now, a lot of people will tell you they take *papaya* enzymes, and I don't see anything wrong with them, but they are fruit enzymes for digestion and not strong enough for cleansing. We have achieved much better results with the plant enzyme Aspergillus oryzae.

Always, the best way for you to get the most from your enzymes is to eat your vegetables and fruits raw and drink your raw vegetable/fruit juices. And get it as close as you can to the way God made it. Unfortunately, we see very few people who eat a totally raw diet, therefore, we are seeing many people who have an imperfect digestive system. It may not be in the right acid/alkaline pH range; it may not have the right enzymes or support the right chemicals and acids the body needs to function. I think the worst thing for the enzymes in the human body is white sugar. Please consider giving up white sugar in any form.

Some people tell me they don't take any white sugar . . . they are drinking diet pop. Well, what do you think that chemical is in there that makes it sweet? True, it's not sugar—*it's worse than the sugar, by far.* If you are going to drink a pop, you are better off drinking the one with sugar than the diet pop with chemical sweeteners. But remember, you are destroying the enzymes in your body, and if you don't have a digestive problem now, *you soon will have!*

Let's concentrate on rebuilding the enzyme "bank" in our bodies, so that the body will have a fighting chance of operating the way it should function.

Here is a little experiment that you can try at home. Get some oatmeal—just the good old kind that grandma used to use—and put some in two different paper cups. Add some warm water to raise the temperature just above normal body temperature, and stir it up. Then take a capsule of enzymes, the ones with all different kinds in it, particularly the amylase which works on the starches/carbohydrates, and stir it into one of the cups. Leave a spoon standing in both cups. Let is set for ½ to 1 hour, then check it out! After about 45 minutes or so, you can pick up the spoon in the cup without the enzymes, and the oats are solid; it's like one great big sucker on a stick . . . it's all stuck together and it now smells sort of like wallpaper paste. But examine the other cup with the enzymes. It will still be soupy and smell just like fresh oatmeal. The difference is that the enzymes have started digesting the oatmeal in their cup. . . they are not particular where they work. If the temperature and pH are right, they begin digesting the food, wherever it is. So, you can do this little experiment and have a lot of fun with it, because we believe that enzymes are a *must* for everybody in this day and age.

An Interview with Michael O'Brien

Michael, I want you to tell me about enzymes, how they help the body, and why we need them, but first, what is an enzyme?

Well, Bud, enzymes are described as a protein, but enzymes actually are the workers in the body. Everything that happens in your body—the biochemical reactions, the digestion, or whatever—has to occur because of an enzyme action. So enzymes are essential. As a matter of fact, Bud, they are so essential that extensive research work that has been done throughout many universities. Dr. Howell (I see you have his book) pulled these studies together and examined them.

When you run out of enzymes, you run out of life. The difference between a man who is alive and a man who is dead is the absence or the breakdown of the enzyme potential. The difference between you and a rock is enzymes.

So, enzymes are absolutely essential. In fact, the body has a metabolic pool of enzymes, but they carry out vital functions. We are supposed to get sufficient enzymes with our nutrition to do the digestive work, and enable our livers to keep renewing our metabolic pool.

Now, I said that enzymes were a protein; actually, enzymes are composed of proteins, and your body uses the enzymes that it has to break down the food that you eat, to supply the nutrients and the proteins necessary (so that it will make more enzymes), to enhance the metabolic pool, and to carry out the vital functions.

If you eat cooked food, the heating destroys the enzymes' ability to do their job. Dr. Howell also pointed out that when you eat cooked food, your body's white blood cell count comes up; that's your defense mechanism. That's the body saying, "You've put something in here that we have no way of handling, or at least a limited method of handling it, so we are going to have to defend ourselves against it."

When you think of these things, you start to realize that nearly everything we eat is cooked. Cooked canned meats actually raise the body's white blood count to the level of poisoning. So, it's just as though you've been poisoned when you eat that. Then you ask yourself the question, "Who eats more of that than anyone else?—who gets that cooked, canned, processed food, like Spam, or canned turkeys and canned hams, and baby foods with meat?" It's these precious little kids who end up getting this kind of food; and no enzymes to handle it, so they become dependent upon their own enzyme pool.

Now, it's important that they have that, except that it's "after the fact." You see, digesting your food after you have a bowel movement is not going to do you any good. We need our enzymes at the "front end" of our digestive processes. When you eat, if you select food that was grown on organic, healthy soil, and you eat it raw, it's going to have an enzyme potential that's phenomenal. And that's what makes the body function properly. Because it's all things in the right time and in the right place.

If your food is digested in the upper (or the cardiac) portion of the stomach, where it is supposed to be digested, then you are going to have a normal total breakdown in the proteins of all the amino acids. As it comes into the low curvature of the stomach, it encounters the hydrochloric acid, which is designed to lower the pH so that the pepsinogen can be converted into pepsin. The pepsin reacts on five amino acids in the low curvature of the stomach, in that acid environment. Of those, one is methianine, which is essential in transporting oxygen to the cell. It's a sulphur-bearing amino acid.

The other three are most essential, and they are so lacking in our body's today that it's phenomenal. . . tryptophane, tyrosine, and phenylalanine. All of them are neuro-transmitting aminos. Now, if those are not reacted upon—if you don't have the polypeptide reaction right away in that acid environment in the low curvature of the stomach— the food passes on into the small intestine, which is an alkaline environment, and you will never have an opportunity for reaction upon that food. You will have missed those essential amino acids. They're gone!

That's why people eat excessively . . . that's why people have problems . . . that's why people end up having putrefactive situations (stagnant, rotting, undigested food) in their colons. And that's an important bottom-line situation. (We'll talk much about putrefaction as we proceed in this discussion.)

In this article about the evidence for intestinal toxemia (you have this, Bud), they are talking about the nature and action of chemicals produced by proteolytic bacteria, and what goes on in the system when you don't properly digest food. The body makes toxins, these bacteria make deadly toxins—endol, phenol, skatol, this type of thing. As in the case of endol, the concentration of phenol in the urine is increased with a high-protein diet. Now, it's not the high-protein diet that increases it, it's the fact that the protein is undigested.

The writer proceeds to discuss the fact that the phenol or the carbolic acid is formed from tyrosine in the process of putrefaction.

Now, if that tyrosine (remember, we talked about those amino acids?) were properly digested in the cardiac portion of the stomach, and then properly reacted upon in the low curvature of the stomach by the pepsin, it would be ready to enter the small intestine (with the alkaline pH), because the acid would have completed its work. You would have no putrefaction.

But trouble starts because people are eating cooked foods with no enzymes, and they no longer chew their food adequately—they don't have to! It's mush, they just suck it down with a negative draft of the esophagus. But the saliva produced in the chewing process is an essential part of the digestive procedure.

Substances formed from putrefaction of undigested tryptophane can lower blood pressure. The tryptomine, from the same source, raises the blood pressure, after an initial depression. So what that's telling us is that if tryptophane is not digested and reacted upon by the pepsin when it gets into your system, it causes all kinds of putrefactive substances with detrimental action. What that means is that it first will lower the blood pressure, and then as it goes through the chemical conversions with the proteolytic bacteria, it will end up raising your blood pressure. Then people take blood pressure medication trying to overcome what's going on from lack of digestion. This goes on all the time.

Anyway, I think that it's important to fully understand that we *must* digest our food, and that is what's so important about taking supplemental enzymes with your meals. As you have the enzymes with the meal, you reduce the amount of undigested proteins, and you quit contributing to the problem.

Now, that doesn't necessarily clean out the

colon, but it quits adding to the problem. And you have methods for cleaning out the colon, Bud; you know what to do for that.

Coming back to what happens. As we said in the beginning, the body is born with an enzyme pool that's limited, the metabolic pool. It is not correct just to say that you have plenty of enzymes, so you don't need to take any more. That's not the answer; you won't have a pool if you don't continue making them. Dr. Howell talked about this "bank account," this enyzme bank account, and he said that you are born with so much, etc. Well, as we studied more and more *The Essentials of Pathophysiology,* by Edward Donovan, we discovered that we, indeed, have a limited pool. The body didn't make just 15 bushel baskets full of enzymes and dump them in there. It made a very limited amount to help you in case of an emergency. It depends upon you functioning in accordance with the laws of nature to continue the body's ability to manufacture the enzymes that it needs. Remember, we said that the enzymes are made out of protein. One of the things you will hear all your life from doctors is that your body makes enzymes, so you don't have to worry about them.

However, they don't address *how* the body makes its own enzymes or what it needs to do that. Well, it has to have digested, utilizable protein in order to achieve that. So, you look at it, and you begin to understand, and you go through all these different things. But invariably you return over, and over, and over again to predigestion (enzymes prior to meals) as the solution.

Then people eat the meat protein, which they can't utilize . . .

. . . because it's heated. Then the lysine is taken out of the food . . . well, it's not exactly *taken out* of the food, but, rather, it is encapsulated when the food is heated. And that encapsulation limits its utilization.

In the article "Nutrition and Food Storage—The Deadly Errors," an excerpt from the book *Famine and Survival in America,* by Howard Ruff, he points out that in limiting amino acids, if a food is even a little low in lysine, according to John Miller, Ph.D., it makes practically worthless the other seven acids as the site of protein formulation. The other seven amino acids are, of course, also essential, but a considerable decline in their availability would be continence without loss of all protein development. On the other hand, a small increase in lysine availability would be wonderfully beneficial, while a small deficit would be disastrous. Now, lysine is an essential.

What they were studying at the time was the nutritional value of the "cookies wafers" they had made to be stored in the bomb shelters back in the 1950's. These cookie wafers had been designed (they thought) to be our sustenance for a long period of time after a nuclear attack. But after they had stocked all these shelters with these things, someone decided perhaps they should *test them* to see if people could live on them.

What they found out was that we didn't need the Russians to do us in; we would do ourselves in by eating the food in the bomb shelters. In their tests, they fed these cookies to rats. The rats in group one who ate regular food did just fine, however, the rats in group two, who were fed these cookies, all died.

So, Dr. Riggs (from the lab) said, "Lysine is not available to my animals. When I check them there is no lysine; they are lysine deficient." The director of the group said that wasn't right. There was lysine. They checked the wafers with chemistry and insisted it was all there.

He said, "But it's heated, and once you heat it you can't get it." So he said, "As the director of the group remarked, 'If you think your chemical tests for availability are good, teach my animals to read your figures,' because they were all dying."

Dependence upon such foods could mean a poor start in life for millions of babies throughout the United States, because we feed them all that baby food.

And we cook it all. . .

We cook it all! So that's the bottom line. On the next page he talks about enzymes and lysines, and how supplementing enzymes liberated that lysine bond once it was located, making it available again. So people are going to ask the question, "What about babies? Can you give enzyme supplements to babies?" And the answer is, "Absolutely! Yes. You betcha'. They need it."

. . . and your pets, and your animals.

You bet! My animals are on enzymes. We look at all these things, and it just comes back over and over again, Bud, to the fact that you must *supply* the enzymes that the body needs. And just this one pamphlet, just this one article, an old one, has more information on the necessity of enzymes than most of the books that have been written. It's blunt, it's right to the point: when you do "this" . . . "this" happens. They dug, found, studied, and learned that we have an enzyme potential that's lost.

Now, yesterday we talked about the aminostatic level of the blood. I thought this was important. Approximately 30% of the population in the United States is overweight. They were discussing why people were overweight, and they are talking here about the aminostatic theory. In studies conducted by Harper and Benevenga, it was shown—both in man and animals—that diets devoid or imbalanced in one or more of the essential amino acids caused abnormal deviations in appetite. And the plasma revealed the absence of one of the essential amino acids. I think it's crucial to understand that people must have a balanced amino acid complex in their system. That's why after a Thanksgiving dinner where one has gorged himself, a half hour later they stand in front of the open refrigerator and just stare. You'll ask what they are looking for, and they'll say that they don't know, they're just hungry. "Well, what are you hungry for?" "I don't know, I'm just hungry."

It's their body telling them they didn't give it what it needs, so they'd better start looking. Well, by the time they finally find it, (the missing aminos) the others have already gone through the system, so they're amino acid deficient.

And they've stripped down the pool of enzymes.

They've wasted it, trying to digest food that was undigestible.

And they've set themselves up for a cause of any disease.

All of them! It's comes right back over and over again, as you know, to the colon, where it all begins. All disease is in the colon . . . no ifs, ands, or buts! This article that I brought in, from which we were just reading, "Evidence for Intestinal Toxemia," is a research paper surveying 165 reputable medical publications. Now, these are not little articles written by some doctor; these are major studies published in recognized journals, such as *The Medical Journal and Record, The New England Journal of Medicine, The Journal of the American Medical Association,* from all major journals.

They asked what were the symptoms of intestinal toxemia: (Now, let's review this again—you get intestinal toxemia because you cannot digest your food. That's where it all originates. It comes from undigested amino acids. They identify it with three; the phenylalanine, the tyrosine, and the tryptophane are the ones which create the greatest putrefactive reaction among the proteolytic bacteria that are there.)

Now, here are the symptoms, and they are really kind of interesting. The first one is allergies. This is a major study. He didn't just say, "Well, we took ten patients and checked them out, and we found that when we detoxified their colon they got over their allergies." There were 472 patients, and he discusses the bacteria and the toxins, *et al,* in the order of the most frequent symptoms, which were endocrine gland disturbances of many types: hypothyroidism, pituitary malfunction, heart disease, hypertension, diabetes, and many others.

Next, he says, "What is another symptom?" Asthma is another symptom of intestinal toxemia, of too much fecal matter lying undigested and putrefying in the colon. Arthritis, cardiac arrhythmias, heart problems come right from the colon. Ear, nose, and throat problems, eclampsia, eye problems, thyroid gland disease, nervous system disorders. (Remember, if you can't get the three aminos that are causing the major problems, it is important to realize that they are the major ones for neurotransmissions.)

Now, if you are not getting the neurotranmissions, you're going to have all these other problems. In other words, how are you going to get the messages to the body so it knows what it's supposed to do?

It just keeps bringing you back again and again to pre-digestion. You have to digest that food. Pre-digestion begins right here in the mouth. Did you know they now have found that there are no food allergies in pre-digested food? If you have a patient who is egg and dairy-allergic, and you pre-digest that food, you can give them milk and egg protein without any problem at all.

Just put some enzymes with it BEFORE they eat it, and that is pre-digesting it?

That's right. Now how does that work in the human body? So that the people reading this book will understand, you begin by putting enzyme-rich food in your mouth and *chewing it* properly (chew each bite slowly and thoroughly, masticating well). People don't chew anymore. They are taught not to chew; they're taught to hurry up and eat, they'll be late for school or work. Everything is just quick, get it down and get done. So they don't chew their food, and it just goes down in big lumps. People don't think they've eaten unless they can feel the lumps going down their throat. All of these things are contributors to sickness and disease, and they've known it for centuries. It's nothing new.

Now, we come down to another experiment. He had his assistant extract a poisonous substance from the feces, which in animal experiments produced quite similar symptoms. The substance was found to be formed by a specific group of bacteria. We are not going to get into that right now, but the important thing was that those undigested proteins, those undigested amino acids that had not been reacted upon, caused a putrefactive condition which gave these bacteria the capacity to react upon them, and that's where you end up with your endol/phenol/skatol, etc.

Some of the mental conditions they reported just from this nervous system disorder were: mental sluggishness (does that sound familiar today?), dullness and stupidity, loss of concentration, (do you know anybody who has that problem?), memory and mental incoordination, irritability, lack of confidence, excessive and useless worry, exaggerated introspection, hypochondria and phobias, depression and melancholy, obsessions and delusions, hallucinations, suicidal tendencies, delirium and stupor. Now, I ask you, does anything in that list sound familiar?

Yes, it does!

So, you go down the line and the schizophrenic substance, the six hydroxic skatol in the urine, was definite evidence that these things were going on in the system. So, senility, low back pain (do you know anybody with low back pain?), it all stems from that toxic colon. They go on to dermatosis (remember, we were talking about this yesterday, and you said to me that they never clean up those

skin disorders until they detoxify the bowel, remember that?)—dermatosis, they proved this
years ago, breast pathology, and cancer. Then he
goes on to say there is no claim that intestinal
toxemia is the cause of cancer, however, some
physicians believe that even the beginning of
malignant disease in various organs comes with
a wide range intestinal stasis.

Do you know how they corrected it here? They
used all different kinds of things, but one of the
main things for getting people over their problems
was they cut their colon out.

You mean they cut it completely out?

No, they remove the section with the putrefaction.

Now they have more problems.

Sure, they have more problems, but they gave
them a reprieve.

*So they took out some of the stuff people should
have been taking out on a fasting and cleanse program anyway.*

That's exactly right. And had they been taking
enzymes, they wouldn't have had that problem in
the first place.

So you're saying that everybody needs enzyme

supplementation at each and every meal?

Oh, and in between meals, too. There are different enzymes you can take between meals to begin restoring that lost enzyme potential [the metabolic pool; the enzymes the body should be producing for emergency purposes].

You don't know which enzymes the people need, so you take them all.

Well, usually you do. And it is possible to identify some of these things. But before I address that, I'm going to reiterate here again the absolute necessity of pre-digesting your food [add supplementary enzymes before eating] or you will be amino-acid deficient. You cannot make the metabolic enzymes. Now, what that causes, so that you have a really clear picture, Bud—and I know you do—is putrefaction in the colon.

Now, what's in the colon goes into the blood stream. The blood takes up that putrefactive substance and transports it to the liver, where the liver manufactures enzymes. So, let's assume that the liver becomes two-thirds full. Then is it correct also to assume that it can be functioning at only one-third of its ability? And if it is functioning at only one-third of its ability, does that mean we are going to be getting only one-third the normal amount of enzymes?

Those enzymes that the liver makes stimulate the endrocine. They are directly related to endocrine function. Did you ever meet a man without a liver?

No.

Did you ever meet a man without a pituitary? I've seen people who only had a seed of it left, just a fragment. But you can't do without the liver because it is a major manufacturing plant. It purifies the system, it manufactures enzymes, it does a lot of things. It stimulates the endocrine.

You see a lot of people today who have a low resistance to disease. This comes right back again to enzymes. There is no getting around it. I know I am being redundant, but if the body can't pre-digest that food, you are going to be amino-acid deficient. And if you are amino-acid deficient, you cannot supply the liver with the protein that it needs to manufacture the metabolic enzymes.

The only time you would not need enzymes is when you eat something like raw honey, which is a pre-digested food, anyhow, so you don't need to take enzymes with that. Anything else, you should, right?

That's true, with certain exceptions. Let's look at something important, because you mentioned the raw honey yesterday and you must be very clear on this. You have to know where that raw honey originated and how it was produced. You are aware that there is only a certain honey that they will give to diabetics; it is the only honey that a diabetic can eat—the tupelo honey. That's because tupelo is the only honey that a bee makes strictly from natural sources—they cannot make tupelo honey from sugar. In the winter, the beekeepers take all the tupelo honey out of the hive and sell it, then they give the bees sugar water. The bee takes the sugar water and makes more honey. Understand that process? Now, they still call that raw honey, but when you eat it you are getting sugar. It's been processed again, and the bees have tried to do something worthwhile with it, but they can't. So, just because they call it "raw" doesn't mean it may not have been made from sugar. You must know the source, and it's always safer to just go ahead and pre-digest it.

Now, you ask me questions. I want you to ask questions that are important to you, Bud, so that you get this down the way you want it, but I think that it's important to understand that people say, "Well, I'm eating raw food; I don't need enzymes."

Wrong!

They have proven in university studies that food grown on mineral-deficient soil is going to be enzyme deficient, even if it is eaten raw and unprocessed. The plant will give off its enzymes to the soil to micronize that soil to get the minerals that it needs in order to survive. So that's an important thing to understand. We need those enzymes.

Then we heat that food and it becomes enzyme deficient, as well as mineral deficient.

You bet! If you read any agricultural book or publication, you are going to find that throughout the United States the soils are deficient in three to five minerals constantly, and it's an increasing deficiency.

So, you look at all of these things, and you begin to understand that many of the things we are doing—no matter how well-intended—are just not wholesome. Even if we are tediously careful about our diet, we likely are not getting the nutrition our bodies require, unless we supplement the diet with vitamins, enzymes, herbs, etc. These deficiencies cause all of the problems we have just covered, and this has been a limited study, but even these few facts are major in their consequences.

There is another thing that is killing off the nutrients and beneficial properties of our fresh produce. Today they're bringing in food from other countries, and everything that is coming into this country in the way of fruits and vegetables is irradiated. They do not allow anything into the country that is not irradiated.

So, you have an enzyme deficit going in. But let's come back to that liver story, because I think the liver story is of particular interest to you. The body will attempt to process the food that you eat, and if it has utilizable protein, it takes it to the liver. There the liver converts it and makes enzymes out of it. Now, if the liver is functioning at only one-third of its capacity (and we made the assumption earlier that possibly you are getting only a third of the enzymes), then your endocrine is going to function at only a third of its capacity. And if it's functioning at only a third of its capacity—if you are getting only a third of your thyroid output— could it be reasonable to assume that you will be functioning at only a third of your capacity. . . that your energy level is going to be down? If your adrenals are only a third, if your thymus is only a third, that your protection has failed?

Fifty-six percent of the digestible protein that you eat will go to the liver, and in the liver it's made into glucose to supply blood sugar. Without that, you are going to be hypoglycemic. Doctors have been fighting this for years and years, but it's a simple thing. Just digest your food and the liver will have protein and the hypoglycemia goes away.

Hypoglycemics who get into enzymes find that it's a tremendous relief. They don't have that two-hour slump where they're looking for a candy bar, a Baby Ruth, or a Dr. Pepper, or something. They say, "Boy, I went from breakfast to lunch, and I didn't have any problem at all. I felt terrific, matter of fact." So these are things that I think are important for people to understand. If your body's not getting the protein, you are going to have hypoglycemia. You may say, "Well, I'm eating the best protein there is." But can you digest it and can you utilize it?

You'll see it in the blood when you can't digest it.

Absolutely! Sure, because it's going to cause putrefactive conditions in the blood, because it's in the colon and the colon affects the blood. Your blood is coming in there, and it's being picked up and all this garbage is being circulated around. People wonder about bad breath, and smelly armpits—you know, deodorant is a major business in the United States, as well as in other parts of the world—but it's because of putrefaction in the colon, being picked by the blood and carried around.

Breath mints! Just think of how many people need breath mints. Even aside from "smoker's breath," just the fact that their colon is causing putrefactive activity that's coming up to the throat is sufficient cause for breath mints or mouth wash. And the bacteria that lives on that stuff migrates. They have a tendency toward an outward migration.

Can you address for us, then, the problem of bacteria in the body, what it does to your blood, then what happens to the bacteria in the blood and in the body.

Well, it depends upon what kind of bacteria it is, Bud. Now the *bad* bacteria, such as E. coli, pseudomonis, and things of that nature, actually get their growth and their start in the system by enzyme-deficient food being undigested, causing that putrefactive condition, and then these bad bacteria start to proliferate. They begin their digestive process by first eating on putrefactive things, until they get going, and then they'll eat anything.

It's just like you. You may not like good food, you may just be a garbage eater. But if you get really, really hungry, a salad is going to taste pretty good to you, because you know you need that to survive. And the intelligence level of bacteria is no less than ours, they just "say," "Whatever I have, I'll use to survive." But it brings you around over and over again to the fact that you need to have enzymes.

Now, we covered the hypoglycemia, we covered the fact that the body makes a pool of enzymes, and we covered the fact that children and babies need enzymes, as well as anyone else. I am asked, "Well, how do you give the enzymes to the baby?" When my children were young, we used to put it in some strawberry jam. And when they had a cold or something, and I was going to give them a little protease to fight the infection, I just put it in a little strawberry jam and gave it to them, because "a spoon full of sugar helps the medicine go down," you know.

You see, protease is a food. People wonder about it and they ask about it. It's food. It's a living thing. It has the capacity to do things. It is a whole food. So is lipase, so is cellulase. In an enzyme complex, you should look for certain things; you should look for protease to digest your proteins. You should look for lipase to digest your fats— now, those are two key factors. You also should look for amylase, because people need amylase. We're heavy starch eaters in this country. And it's because when you can't digest protein, then your

body says, "Well, I'd better start digesting starch."
So you are hungry for starch; you need bread, you
need carbohydrates, you have to have them to
bring that blood sugar up.

Because if there is no amylase...

...you can't get them. So, when you are depleted of protease, you start on the amylase. And
when you are depleted of amylase, then you go
after the lipase, the fats.

Now, let's watch this as a scenario. If you can't
digest your food, you can't get the protein, and
you are going to become protease deficient, protein deficient...that means you are going to
become hypoglycemic.

Now, this scenario will give you an idea what's
going to happen over the long haul. The blood
sugar is not being maintained—you're hypoglycemic. At that point, you say, "What's the next
stage?" The next stage is, "Well, I have to digest
carbohydrates—starches." So, your body starts in
on that...until you deplete that enzyme resource.

First, you went through a period of time when
all you had was the hypoglycemic reaction. You
ate the candy bar, blood sugar went up, two hours
later it was down, so you were eating something
else. You're up and down and up and down. Now
the body says, "We're out of those amylase enzymes, we're not getting all we need of those, so
what are we going to do?" Now, you have a deficiency symptom, so you start using the lipase-

related foods, therefore, fat becomes your preferential diet. You need the fat, you need the butter, you need this, you need that.

Now what are you into? You're into a diabetic situation. So, a hypoglycemic condition, left uncorrected, may evolve into diabetes.

What about PMS? You see the woman who has PMS is not getting protein, she's not capable of transporting calcium, she's not making hormones, and she has PMS. And what is she going to be? She may end up being the woman who has osteoporosis.

It's like a chain reaction. . . it starts in one place and, if not corrected, will end up in another. So, when you look at these scenarios, you want to know what you can do to break the chain. You need an enzyme protease to digest your protein. You need amylase to digest your starches. You need lipase to digest your fats. You need cellulase. The body doesn't make cellulase. All of the studies that were ever done for cancer used raw fiber. It has cellulase in it.

Cellulase is a gutwall transporter and is essential in the body; without it, how are you going to break down fiber? The answer is, "You can't." Nature designed it to be there. And doctors say not to worry about enzymes because your body makes them. Well, that may have been the way God designed it (before we messed up everything), but your body requires all those major ingredients to continue making them.

Another question many doctors ask is, "Are they

habit forming." And I reply, "Well, absolutely, they are habit forming. God put them into the food for our body." Enzymes are not habit forming in the sense that they are implying, you can quit them any time you like. We did that before...

But you're right back to disease!

You're right back to disease. Over and over again.

God created enzymes in every living food. And we're not talking here about a differential in pre-amorphic being creation or evolution; this is all creation. God created everything. But in your body, some of the preamorphic conditions transfer because your body is trying to compensate and adjust for not having what it needs.
And it does, it actually does a tremendous job on that. You're right. But it's only going to do that for so long, then you wear it out. And science is proving that right now.
Today, as we sit here and talk, it is the 26th of June 1993—did you know that you are 98% different right now than you were the 26th of June last year? 98% of the cells of your body are totally different cells, totally renewed. They're not the same cell that was there, even the hard bone structure has changed. The calcium has been lifted up and more calcium put down. And the cells and everything have changed.
And we ask ourselves why we are aging, why

we are deteriorating, why we are having these problems. Well, it's because we are not giving the body the enzymes and the nutrients that it needs to carry out the functions to maintain itself. At any given time, your body is no more than three years old. Think of it! They used to say seven years. Now they have brought it down to three because they have watched it occur. But they knew years ago—it was common knowledge—that your body was never any older than seven years of age. And today you're down to three.

So why do we get old, and get ill, and get all these degenerative conditions? It's because of our lifestyle. People say, "How long to I have to take these enzymes. Do I have to take these forever." I tell them, "No. You don't have to take them forever, just through this lifetime. Maybe the next time around, we'll be more intelligent!"

You have to take them as long as you want to feel good. As long as you can't get them out of your food, because the Garden of Eden had plenty of enzymes in everything, and it was unpolluted.

That's right. Absolutely. No ifs, ands, or buts about it . . . it was there.

So, you begin to consider the different situations that occur and ask, "How do I know when I need one particular type of enzyme?" You need them all. I could say that protease was related to infections and viral conditions, and that you could take protease and it works really well for that, but what difference does that make?

I could talk to you about lipase, and I could tell you that a diabetic on lipase can start to bring down their insulin requirement. There was a truck driver who had lost his license—that was his living. He made his living driving trucks. He was diabetic, and as long as he was on oral insulin, the state let him retain his license. But as soon as his diabetes got bad enough to require injections, they pulled his license, on the premise that if he were driving down the road and suddenly needed that injection, he could have a bad accident. So they took his license away, and this guy was devastated because he didn't know anything else. He asked me what to do. I told him if he started digesting his food and added a little extra lipase to his life, he would begin to digest the fat.

You remember we discussed this; you go from inability to digest protein, then you digest starch, then you digest fat, in your progression from hypoglycemia to diabetes. In every case of diabetes, you invariably will find ketodes in the urine. Every time! It's because that's what your body is digesting, what it's breaking down. It took the truck driver about four months, but he was off of his injections and got his license back. He really was happy, because he got his job back and had a way to make a living again.

You can talk about amylase being important to the person who has hives and swelling and ends up with allergic reactions to bee stings, poison ivy, poison oak, and things of this nature, and it works

. . . it works every time. But I think the important thing is that anytime you talk to people about enzymes, they must realize that they need them all. They need to look at the sugar enzymes (the enzymes that were removed from pure cane sugar by C & H) so that they can digest them and put them into activity.

Could you share with us your goals in life. I know you are doing the Lord's work all the time, but I would like you to tell us in this book what you consider the Lord's work, as you see it.

I was raised in a Christian family. I went through my rebellion, but I read, I read the Bible continuously. There was an interesting statement by Christ when He was here 2,000 years ago. He said that the laws of God are written in the heart of man, and God's temple is not a temple made by hands. I used to wonder about that, then I came to realize that your body is the temple of the Holy Spirit. And there are a lot of Scriptures in there that tell us that God will not dwell in an unclean temple, so I started working on cleaning up mine. If my temple is the dwelling place, then you know where the kingdom of heaven is located? It is within. And if the kingdom of heaven is within, then that is where God dwells, and it says God will not dwell in an unclean temple.

So, I've dedicated my life, Bud, as you probably have heard me say before, to rebuilding the temples of the living God, to setting them up, to making them so that they function the way God designed them to function. And my prayer every day is that God will show me the structure of that temple, so that I will know how to rebuild it, and then that He will make available without any restraints—because that is His promise—all the building materials. He said He would supply our every need. Now, that may require intelligence on our part in order to preserve it, but He will make it available to us if we have the intelligence to function. It's just like He's made life and health available to us if we are willing to do what it takes.

But you can't serve two masters, and we can't be out here happily living like the rest of the people...

...*on coffee and doughnuts, hamburgers and pop*...

...that's right, and expect Him to bless us and have a good wholesome temple. It just doesn't work, so I dedicated my life to rebuilding the temples of God, and my prayer is to accomplish that.

I may touch the lives of only a few thousand people, but in touching the lives of a few thousand people, I hope that they have the courage and devotion to do the same thing...touch the lives of a few thousand people. They call that chain reaction, but that's good. We can change the world that way.

That's wonderful, Michael. I certainly appreciate

*this interview, and I know that those who read this
book will benefit from this critical information.*

Chapter 8

Nutrition According to God's Word

Unless noted otherwise, all scriptures are from the New King James Version of the Holy Bible.

Some of you have been so sick that you have cried out in desperation, "God, I need a miracle!" How do we get sick, and where does it originate? Are some of us just meant to be sick, while others remain healthy all their life? And why are some people healed miraculously and others never seem to receive the miracle they so badly need?

God's Word has much to say about health and healing, miracles and living in continuous good health. When we know and understand what the Word of God tells us, we can apply those promises to our lives with confidence.

If you have asked the question, "How do I receive a miracle when I am in need of one?" you are not alone. This is a question that I'm sure has plagued mankind since the Words were penned under the anointing of the Holy Spirit.

But of one thing we have assurance . . . the abundance of scriptures dealing with the subject make it perfectly clear that God wants us healthy, and if we are not, He wants to heal us.

> *Beloved, I wish above all things that thou mayest prosper and be in health, even as thy soul prospereth.*
> III John 2 (KJV)

> *. . . for I am the Lord that healeth thee.*
> Exodus 15:25 (KJV)

> *Bless the Lord, O my soul: and all that is within me, bless His holy name. . . . who healeth all thy diseases; . . . .*
> Psalm 103:1-3 (KJV)

In fact, God not only wants us physically healthy, but spiritually and emotionally healthy, as well.

> *He heals the broken-hearted and binds up their wounds.*   Psalm 147:3

However, the thrust of this book will address primarily the physical aspects of achieving good health.

It seems like stating the obvious to point out that living in divine health is always better than relying upon divine healing. Divine health was God's plan for mankind, and there is no mention of sickness prior to the sin of Adam and Eve; in fact, we are told that the creation was "very good" and that they had dominion over all the creation.

I believe the Bible indicates that some folks are sick because of sin, but it also tells us that this is not always the case. Remember when Jesus was asked who sinned, the man or his parents, and His answer was neither? One example to consider is found in Micah 6:13:

> Therefore also will I make thee sick in smiting thee, in making thee desolate because of thy sins. (KJV)

Now, sin is not the only reason for sickness (at least not the individual's sin—even though sickness entered with original sin). There are many believers living holy, righteous lives, yet they suffer disease and illness in their bodies. Why?!? Even though they may not be sinning intentionally, they are unwittingly abusing their bodies, the temple of the Holy Spirit.

> Know ye not that ye are the temple of God and that the Spirit of God dwelleth in you? If any man defile the temple of God,

him shall God destroy; for the temple of
God is holy, which temple ye are.
                    I Corinthians 3:16,17 (KJV)

You are the caretaker of the temple, and even
though we are not to worship the temple, neither
are we to abuse it. Everything from improper nutrition to stress and overwork takes a toll on our
physical bodies, and many times on our mental
state, as well. And until you have examined yourself (as is recommended before we receive Communion), don't rule out the possibility of unconfessed sin in your life. Receiving Communion
"unworthily" is another reason given for having
"many sick among you, and some even sleep [are
dead]."

That is why a man should examine him-
self carefully. . . . For if he eats the bread
and drinks from the cup unworthily . . . he
is trifling with the death of Christ. That is
why many of you are weak and sick, and
some have even died.
                    I Corinthians 11:28-30 (LB)

Later in this chapter we will investigate some
of the biblical references dealing specifically with
eating habits, cleansing habits, and a number of
the *thou shalt's* and the *thou shalt not's*. But before
we get into that, there are a couple of points I would
like to call to your attention, then I will share with
you how I go about an average day, so far as my

nutrition and supplements are concerned.

Sometimes people haven't suffered enough yet to make them willing to undertake a healthy regimen, which, in the case of most individuals, probably will require reexamining your entire life-style and establishing all new priorities regarding your eating habits, work patterns, spiritual growth, etc. If people are in apparent good health, in addition to being somewhat ignorant concerning the real facts about nutrition, they most likely will ignore or put off the physical cleansing and nutritional needs of their bodies . . . but if they become ill—especially with something for which the medical community can offer little or no help—they suddenly can get real serious about doing something to help their body rid itself of the ailments. Unfortunately, many times it is a case of "too little, too late." Fortunately, God designed our bodies to renew and regenerate themselves, given the proper cleansing and nutrition, so many people are helped, even though health professionals and others have given up on them.

God made man a free agent, with the option to choose what he wants to do; however, the right to choose does not come without a price. We always must live with the consequences of our choices. This isn't some sort of Divine trick God played on mankind. Even after he ate of the forbidden fruit, God gave man "laws" and "commandments"—in other words, instructions to help him make the *right* decisions with his divinely permitted ability to "choose."

There were "instructions" give to Adam and Eve
in the Garden of Eden, and again to Noah . . . these
are referred to as Covenants. But the ones with
which we are most familiar were given by God to
Moses for the children of Israel and currently are
called the Ten Commandments. These were followed by more detailed regulations concerning
diet and cleanliness (in the book of Leviticus),
which were established to keep the children of
Israel well-nourished, disease-free, and free of
plagues.

Jesus said He didn't come to do away with the
Law, but to fulfill it. Therefore, even though we
live today under grace, we must remember that
God thought it important enough to tell us twice
(through the apostle Paul):

*All things are lawful for me, but all things
are not helpful [or expedient]. . . .*
                    I Corinthians 6:12; 10:23

And when taken in full context, both of these scriptures refer to food.

The Holy Spirit should flow from you like a pure,
clean river, without having to emanate from a dirty
body. We are to be vessels made for the Potter's
use, and not the kind Jesus described when he
accused the Pharisees of being all clean and pol-
ished on the outside, but full of filth inside (Matthew 23:25,26). That illustration may be taken
both spiritually and physically. And you first must
clean up your own life before you can be a truly

effective servant who God wants to use to minister health and healing to others, not just spiritually, but physically, as well.

The Bible tells us that without faith, it is impossible to please God. Faith is an active word, not a passive one. I like to describe faith as acting on what I believe. And having put my faith into actions, then I stand on God's Word that tells me:

> *No weapon formed against you shall prosper;....*   Isaiah 54:17

You know, folks, it doesn't matter whether you choose to cleanse now or later, but think how much more you can accomplish for the kingdom of God if you are truly healthy. Consider the following points.

1. For a clean spirit, you need God's Holy Spirit.
2. For a clean body, you need a bath, inside as well as outside.

You actually can have each cell in your body clean, but that takes time and determination.

The Author's Daily Routine and Nutrition

I want to share with you my personal daily regimen. It does not mean that everyone will be the same, but it is what I must do to maintain my own health.

I start my day with six or seven of the Pro Guard

Plus, which is the S.O.D. Super Oxide Dismutase. These are taken upon rising, and I don't eat or drink anything for 30 minutes, which allows it to get into my system and be absorbed into my blood before I take in any food. I believe everyone should have three or four of these, but I feel that in order for me to build my immune system the way I should, I take seven every morning.

Later in the morning when I have my first juice, I will take at least two Spirulina Pacifica. These supply the trace minerals or elements, as well as the beta carotene which I need. Lots of times people will need at least four of these, twice a day. The reason is that we are no longer getting the proper nutrients out of our food, and this is a perfect food.

So my day begins with antioxidants and blue-green algae (Spirulina). The first juice I give my body each morning is a combination of carrot/apple/vegetable. I don't like eating a lot of raw vegetables, therefore, I juice my broccoli, asparagus, zucchini, and all the others. I put in about 20% greens (I don't use just one or two, I use a wide variety of greens), 10% apple, and the greatest portion of the remainder is carrots, along with some beet juice.

I find that drinking beet juice is an excellent test to determine if you are absorbing what you are eating. What you are *putting into* your body isn't nearly as important as what it can *absorb*. Add beet juice to your drink, then watch your next stool. If it is "beet red," then your body is not absorbing your food, it is passing right on through, gaining very few nutrients. When your body is properly absorbing what it is given, then you won't see the beet juice in the stool. The amount you spend on expensive foods and supplements is of no benefit to you if your body is not absorbing them.

At the time of my first meal, I take at least three of the Bio-Energy 321A enzymes, then regardless of what I put into my stomach, the enzymes are there and ready to go to work aiding the digestive process. For years my body was absolutely bankrupt of enzymes because everything I ate was cooked, and there are no enzymes in cooked foods. In addition, I take the following supplements daily: Vitamin A, Vitamin B, Vitamin C, Vitamin E, Zinc, Magnesium, Potassium, and a multilevel vitamin and mineral combination. These are the things my body needs to maintain good health.

There is another thing that I believe everyone needs; it is Chromium Picolinate. Because of many years of eating sugar, one develops a sugar intolerance, and if you are borderline diabetic or hypoglycemic, for goodness sake, take the Chromium Picolinate because it will help you.

Here is what I should be eating: six vegetables every day, two fruits, one carbohydrate, and one protein. I don't intentionally eat any fat, other than what little may be in the food that I eat. Personally, I don't believe we need any fat; even the Bible tells us not to eat the fat.

Normally, I have my first solid food about 2:00

to 3:00 p.m. My first juice is usually vegetable, because that is alkaline and is what my body's cells need first. Then later on, about midday, I'll have a fruit juice, which is something that I really like, followed by my main meal (2:00 to 3:00 p.m.), and vegetable juice again about 5:00 or 6:00 p.m. I no longer drink anything with my meals. I used to be one of those who had to wash everything down, but no more. I drink either one-half hour before the meal or one and a half hours after the meal. And I find that I don't drink as much water as I used to drink, because the juices are full of nutrition and satisfying my sense of thirst or the craving I had for water before.

Like everyone else, I frequently want to eat something before going to bed, so I'll put a couple of bananas in the blender, along with some other fruit in season (or if it's winter, something we put in the freezer when it was in season), and blend it all together. Then I'll drink a glass or glass and a half before I go to bed. It's very nice to have this at bedtime, because your stomach is full and you have that sense of satisfaction—you feel like you just got through eating a meal.

There is another thing that I need, and I'll probably need it for the rest of my life. I need fiber, because for so many years I ate so much cooked food and had so much constipation, that my colon is sluggish. On a daily basis before I go to bed, I usually take with my last drink anywhere from two to four of the L. Salivarius friendly bacteria. I do this because I still have a sluggish, partly prolapsed colon from so many years of not keeping it empty and clean. In other words, my colon sags down. So if I do not keep it empty and clean, it starts getting heavier and heavier, putting pressure on the organs below, and I actually can feel the pressure it applies. I don't like that feeling, so I keep it clean now.

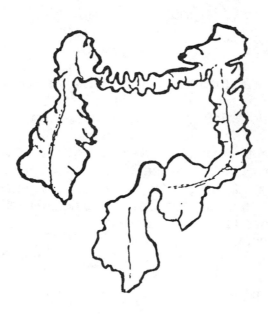

The average length of time for food to pass from your mouth to your stool should be from 12 to 18 hours. If every meal you eat is cooked and contains meat, it could be as long as 96 to 100 hours before it becomes stool. If that is the case, you need more help, i.e. fiber, to move the food on through.

Finally, I'd refer you back to Psalm 103:5, which is an excellent scripture.

> *Who satisfies your mouth with good things, so that your youth is renewed like the eagle's.*   Psalm 103:5

Now, I take a little literary license in interpreting this verse, and I recognize that this may not be the actual interpretation intended, but I like to think of it this way. The eagle appears to be ageless; he doesn't seem to grow old and weak; he soars until it is his time to die. I think that if I put in my mouth only the "good things" to which the scripture refers, then I, too, can soar (be in good health) until my life comes to its natural end.

Another couple of scriptures to which I would like to call your attention are found in Daniel 1:8 and 12. Daniel and his three friends were the first reported vegetarians.

> *But Daniel purposed in his heart that he would not defile himself with the portion of the king's delicacies, nor with the wine which he drank; . . . . "Please test your servants for ten days, and let them give us*

vegetables to eat and water to drink. Then let our countenances be examined before you, and the countenances of the young men who eat the portion of the king's delicacies; and as you see fit, so deal with your servants."
                                    Daniel 1:8,12-13

I'm not a true vegetarian. I eat fish; I enjoy salmon a few times a year, as long as it is fresh, and other fish, as long as it is deep running, ocean or lake, cold water, with gills, scales, and fins—I really enjoy it. However, I do try to limit my intake, even of good fish, because if I indulge myself too often, it also will affect my health.

I have another personal problem . . . my system will not retain sodium, so I must address this need, as well. Therefore, I take one or two capsules of Whex, which is a powdered form of goat's whey. Goat's whey is the highest known source of natural sodium, and the body can utilize it. So I don't use salt on my food, but I do use Whex when I feel that it does need some seasoning, because my body readily can absorb sodium in that form.

I don't expect you to follow my own personal program. I'm just sharing it with you to give you some basics. Each person's body is different, therefore, each needs their own basic plan. The bodies were probably the same in the beginning, but what each of us has done to our own body since we were born means that they are probably very different now.

I like the old saying that a lady told me once a while back, that *she was sick and tired of being sick and tired!* So I go on the colonic board once a week just to keep the toxins flowing out of my body and maintain a clean intestine. On the day that I go on the board, I do a one-day juice fast, using only fresh juice that I make myself. Since I travel a lot, I find that I can get up early, make all my drinks for the day, and put them in the car in an ice chest and drink them throughout the day as needed. Your stomach may think your throat's been cut, but that's all in your head . . . you really won't starve. So a travel day is a very good day to fast.

But you'll find that life is a lot more pleasant if you can work out your own program. To me, this is not a diet, it's a way of life, because I've learned to love this program. I don't call it a diet, because *diet* is a bad word. To me, it's *life.* And that's the way I want to live the rest of my life. Another precious little thought to me is that the flower grows to get out of the dirt, and that's what you and I must do . . . grow to get out of the dirt.

Nutrition from the Bible

The Bible is full of scriptures about health, healing, and eating habits, most of which are self-explanatory. So I just want to make you aware of a number of these, with limited comments. But before I begin, I want to call to your attention one thing in particular. Often when the Bible refers to *meat,* it means your daily food, not the flesh of an animal, fish, or fowl, unless specifically indicated to be such.

Vegetables, Fruits, Herbs, Seeds—Hybrids

> *And God said, "See, I have given you every herb that yields seed which is on the face of all the earth, and every tree whose fruit yields seed; to you it shall be for food."*
> Genesis 1:29

We are to eat seeds (grains) which are capable of reproducing their own kind, season after season. Hybrids are not able to do that; you have to replant with new seed each year. Farmers grow hybrid corn and other crops because it produces a greater yield; however, it produces much less nutrients. In fact, if you fed your farm animals nothing else, they soon would grow weak and eventually die. So if you eat only hybrids, you are depriving yourself of the nutrition your body needs (and you think you are getting by eating the proper foods).

Fish—Fins and Scales

> *These you may eat of all that are in the water: whatever in the water has fins and scales, whether in the seas or in the rivers—that you may eat. . . . Whatever in the water does not have fins or scales —that shall be an abomination to you.*
> Leviticus 11:9,12

Fat and Blood

> *And the Lord spoke to Moses, saying,*
> *"Speak to the children of Israel, saying:*
> *'You shall not eat any fat, of ox or sheep*
> *or goat. . . . Moreover you shall not eat*
> *any blood in any of your dwellings, wheth-*
> *er of bird or beast."*   Leviticus 7:22-26

Life Is in the Blood

> *. . . for it is the life of all flesh. Its blood*
> *sustains its life. Therefore I said to the chil-*
> *dren of Israel, "You shall not eat the blood*
> *of any flesh, for the life of all flesh is its*
> *blood. Whoever eats it shall be cut off."*
> Leviticus 17:14

Abstain from Blood

> *. . . but that we write to them to abstain*
> *from things polluted by idols, from sexual*
> *immorality, from things strangled, and*
> *from blood.*   Acts 15:20

There are many scriptures that warn us against
eating the blood, and the reasons are not just spiritual. Because the life literally is in the blood, there
are strong physiological reasons for that command,
as well. As the body uses fuel in metabolism, each
cell gives off a byproduct (toxin/waste) as a result
of doing its work. These toxins are carried in the

bloodstream from each cell to the kidneys, which excretes them in the form of urine. So if you are drinking/eating the blood of the meat, you are drinking the urine (toxins). Now, I know that sounds horrible, but that's the way it is.

Do All to the Glory of God

> *Therefore, whether you eat or drink, or whatever you do, do all to the glory of God.*   I Corinthians 10:31

We are to eat to the glory of God, not to the glory of our flesh—which may "crave" something even if it's bad for us. Your blood will make your body crave what you have conditioned it to believe it needs to survive. If you feed it an abundance of soft drinks, coffee, candy bars, French fries, and hot fudge sundaes, you will physically crave those things for awhile when your body does not get them.

Revising Habits Begins with a Willing Mind

> *For if there is first a willing mind. . . .*
> II Corinthians 8:12

Rest—An Essential for Good Health, Spiritually and Physically

> *"Come to Me, all you who labor and are heavy laden, and I will give you rest. Take*

*My yoke upon you and learn from Me, for
I am gentle and lowly in heart, and you will
find rest for your souls."*
                                    Matthew 11:28,29

Our bodies need an adequate amount of rest to
remain healthy, in addition to the spiritual rest described in the scripture above. God has ordained
that mankind should work only from sunup to
sundown, six days a week, resting on the seventh.
"Burning the candle at both ends" was never God's
intent for us, and it's harmful to both our physical
and mental well-being. (Read Genesis 2:2,3 and
Exodus 20:9 ff.) Do you know that the only reason
we have "weeks" on our calendar is because God
ordained six days of work and one day of rest? The
other divisions all are related to the heavenly
bodies in some way, i.e. the earth revolves once
(a day), the moon goes around it (a month), it goes
around the sun (a year), but not the concept of the
"week." Yet, it is found in every culture, no matter
how remote or primitive, but no one knows why
because there is no astronomical reason for it . . . it
just exists. God established it at creation, Noah
carried it through the Flood, and Moses was given
it again for the children of Israel in the Ten Commandments. Did God need to rest after speaking
everything into creation and making man? I think
not. He did so as a pattern for the way his creation
was designed to live.

By the way, vacations also are recommended.

Jesus advocated and lived out the pattern for us to "come away" from the cares of life for a little while for a time of refreshing. And remember David's green pastures where God made him to lie down?

Fasting and Prayer for Cleansing, Spiritually and Physically

"However, this kind does not go out except by prayer and fasting."
Matthew 17:21

Jesus is referring in this passage to spiritual cleansing, specifically casting out demons; however, physical cleansing is achieved by using much the same methods.

Fasting and Prayer Among the Elders

So when they had appointed elders in every church, and prayed with fasting, they commended them to the Lord in whom they had believed.   Acts 14:23

Fasting is a method of cleansing the physical body from within, as well as a spiritual endeavor when accompanied by prayer. Read Leviticus Chapters 11 through 15 to find out all about the cleansing and health codes established for the children of Israel. The cleansing recommended in this book is mild when compared with the stringent requirements spelled out in Leviticus.

Keeping His Commandments

> *Now by this we know that we have Him, if we keep His commandments. He who says, "I know Him," and does not keep His commandments, is a liar, and the truth is not in him. But whoever keeps His word, truly the love of God is perfected in him. By this we know that we are in Him.*
> I John 1:3-6

Many of us want to be "Cafeteria Christians." That is, we like to pick and choose which commandments to obey. If we expect to enjoy the benefits of good health, then we should "choose" to obey the laws in God's Word governing what we should eat and how it should be prepared. I am not speaking here in contradiction to the Word which tells us it is what comes out of a man that defiles him, not what goes in. That refers to spiritual defilement; but if we willfully disobey God's instructions about what is expedient for us (even though all things may be lawful), then we are defiling our physical bodies, and there are many admonitions in the Word against doing that.

Nothing is Impossible

> *For with God nothing will be impossible.*
> Luke 1:37

If all things are possible with God, and we truly believe we are born-again sons and daughters of God, then we have no excuse for not restructuring our habits to align with God's instructions regarding our eating and cleansing, or for believing God for healing if we need it. . . except for a lack of faith. And there are plenty of scriptures to help us deal with that problem, as well.

Forgiveness and Healing

> *Who forgives all your iniquities, Who heals all your diseases, Who redeems your life from destruction. . . .*   Psalm 103:3,4

Carrying strife and unforgiveness in your heart is one of the best ways I know to bring on illness and disease. We are to forgive those who offend us if we expect to be forgiven—Jesus makes that clear. According to God's pattern (above), He forgives, then heals, then redeems from destruction. If you harbor bitterness and unforgiveness, get rid of it! It's the first step toward good physical health.

Dining with the Lord Who Heals

> *. . . If you diligently heed the voice of the Lord your God and do what is right in His sight, give ear to His commandments and keep all His statutes, I will put none of the diseases on you. . . . For I am the Lord who heals you.*   Exodus 15:26

You have a choice 21 times a week to decide whether you are going to eat with God or eat with the devil. If I told you to take two to five pounds of medicine every day, you'd think I was crazy, but you take in two to five pounds of food every day. I believe this makes it clear that your food should be your medicine, and your medicine should be your food.

Divine Peace vs. Heart Trouble and Fear

> *Peace I leave with you. My peace I give to you; not as the world gives do I give to you. Let not your heart be troubled, neither let it be afraid.*   John 14:27

In another scripture it talks about men's hearts failing them for fear (Luke 21:26). This clearly illustrates that emotional conditions will have physical results. Put your trust in the Lord, who gives perfect peace—even in troubled and stressful times. Learn to live in confidence, dwelling in safety in the presence of God, as described in Psalm 91 which says that no evil shall befall you, nor shall any plague come near your dwelling (vs. 10), and He will give His angels charge over you to keep you in all your ways . . . they shall bear you up in their hands, lest you dash your foot against a stone (vss. 11 and 12).

The Sin Question

*As far as the east is from the west, so
far has He removed our trangressions [sins]
from us.*   Psalm 103:12

Many of us are sick as a result of sin in our life,
and many just as a result of reaping the crop of
wild oats we sowed in our youth, but that does not
mean God will not hear our prayer and restore our
youth "as the eagle's." In fact, just above this scripture (vs. 12) in verse 10 we read, "He has not dealt
with us according to our sins, nor punished us
according to our iniquities." And in Joel 2:25,26
we are told: "So I will restore to you the years that
the locusts have eaten. . . . You shall eat in plenty
and be satisfied, and praise the name of the Lord
your God, who has dealt wondrously with you. . . ."
Therefore, we are never too old to ask God's forgiveness and begin to reshape our habits. And one
more warning: old habits die hard, so don't give
up when you fail (and you will!), just keep trying
with a sincere heart to do the right thing for your
body, and God will help you to improve your ways.

It is reported in Acts 20:24 about finishing the
race; also in I Timothy 4:7 ". . . I have fought the
good fight, I have finished the race, I have kept
the faith." So, "let us be not weary in well-doing,
for in due season we shall reap if we faint not [don't
give up] (Galatians 6:9 and II Thessalonians 3:13).

The body is like a great orchestra. You can
orchestrate your body with vitamins, minerals,

herbs, and enzymes, but that's only a Band-aid, unless you have cleansed the body. When you begin caring for your body correctly, you can orchestrate it to a state of homeostasis, where every cell and organ is working in harmony as God designed it, to make your body a living temple. At your invitation, God will live in the temple and you can be at harmony with Him . . . that's the only way to have peace and health, living a life with your Lord Jesus Christ.

A long time ago, the prophet Hosea wrote under the inspiration of the Holy Spirit, "My people are destroyed for a lack of knowledge . . ." (Hosea 4:6). His warning is a warning for us today.

Chapter 9

God's Plagues—Treating Drug-Resistant Diseases

Many times in medicine—because the full name may be particularly cumbersome or just from the frequency of use—the acronym of a disease or treatment (the first letter of each word or syllable) becomes better known than the disease which the letters represent.

One such example much in use today, and becoming better known all the time, is DRS which is the acronym for a **D**rug **R**esistant **S**train of viruses, many now reaching epidemic proportions. There is a lot of debate about how a strain becomes drug-resistant, but I have some personal thoughts on the subject.

In my opinion, the problem originated in some of the third-world countries who have been dispensing a variety of antibiotics across the counter to the general populace, without benefit of the control, counsel, and instruction in their proper use by a qualified physician. Whenever someone's child would get the sniffles, cold, or flu, rather than using the old-fashioned remedies, they just would go down to the local pharmacy and get a supply of the latest, most potent antibiotic available.

They use these antibiotics freely, without seeking a doctor's care. . . and frequently. When they feel better, they stop taking them, whereas a doctor would prescribe that they take them long after they start feeling better, because all the germs are not yet dead. The disease is driven "underground"; it appears to be gone, but really isn't, and many suffer relapses.

In other cases, the germs that have no natural immunity to the antibiotic are killed, leaving behind only those with a natural immunity to that particular form of antibiotic, who then pass around that immunity to the others as they safely multiply over a period of time.

Now the people from the third-world countries (who have developed in their bodies diseases which are immune to antibiotic treatment) are immigrating to the United States and other developed nations, bringing with them these DRS (drug-resistant strains) of diseases.

Today, there is good evidence that some of these diseases can no longer be cured by the antibiotics that used to work on them (TB is a good example). In my opinion, this can be traced back to the abuse of the antibiotics. It takes a pharmaceutical company about twelve to fourteen years to develop a drug that is useful against a particular virus, properly test it for effectiveness and safety, then put it on the market.

Now, it is not widely publicized in the media (for obvious reasons), but I understand that TB (tuberculosis) has now reached epidemic proportions across the United States, and that they have nothing on the market. . . repeat: *nothing*. . . that is effective in the treatment of this particular strain. They can't kill it! So in many states, particularly in the poverty-stricken sections of large metropolitan areas, TB already has reached the epidemic stage. It would take considerable time to develop an effective antibiotic for this strain of TB.

Then consider the deadly Hanta virus which appeared recently on an Indian reservation in the southwest U.S. (and an isolated case in The Dalles, Oregon). It took a long time for the Center for Disease Control to identify it, and even longer to figure out how they got it. It turns out that it was caused by the waste from infected deer mice and rats, leaving their urine and droppings in the dust and streams. Of course, there is no known cure. And the concensus seems to be that these animals had their origin in the orient, where this virus has been known for many years. Many third-world nations have a myriad of bacteria, germs, viruses, parasites, etc. not yet known in our nation, but with the "shrinking" globe, it is only a matter of time before we have to deal with more and more illnesses for which we have no effective medical treatment.

Below I will list several with which we already are familiar, but because space is limited I will give only brief mention to each one.

AIDS is the one that has reached epidemic proportions around the globe, and the one that currently is receiving the greatest amount of attention. That doesn't even include all those who are considered HIV-positive and likely will come down with full-blown AIDS in the future, making this plague even more deadly and costly. Yet, in spite of the millions and millions of dollars put into research, and all the political pressure being brought to bear, science still seems very far from coming up with any drug that shows even remote signs of curing AIDS. In fact, the scientific community probably would be ecstatic if they just could find a way to immunize against catching it, even if they could do nothing to help those who already have contracted the disease. . . at least that would put control of the disease in sight sometime in the foreseeable future.

Not long ago, we had an epidemic in Milwaukee because of a parasite that got into the drinking water and failed to die in the chlorine and bromine that had been added to make the water safe to drink (apparently the chemical mix was incorrect). The parasite was cryptosporidium parvum. Two thousand people were affected by severe diarrhea and other stomach disorders. One person died and five others succumbed to fatal diseases after drinking the water.

Also communities in Georgia, Texas, Pennsylvania, and Oregon have been affected by this parasite (or others). The parasites are carried by mammals, particularly young livestock. As we get more and more pollution, it can be in your lakes and rivers, or anything else, eventually making its way into your water supply or other surface areas where you may come into contact with it.

There are other parasites in the back country, especially where you find infected beaver, who spread a parasite called Giardia. But in cities, many varieties are carried by rats. A magazine recently reported an outbreak of kidney disease in Baltimore, Maryland, as a result of rats. The study covered more than 8,000 people there. They referred to a similar Asian origin as the Hanta virus, but this one caused a hemorrhaging of the kidney, and many Baltimore hospitals are reporting patients with apparent kidney disease, which, in fact, is of parasitic origin.

This crop of epidemics seems to have begun about the time we had the outbreak of Legionnaire's Disease. The symptoms appeared to be like pneumonia, but were caused by a bacteria that had developed in the cooling tower of the air conditioning systems, and was being vaporized and pumped right into the air they were breathing. The same bacteria also is found in lakes, ponds, streams, puddles, and compost piles.

I believe there are going to be more and more of these "plagues," if that's what you choose to call them, and as our personal immune system becomes weaker and weaker, it will not be able to fight off the invading bacteria, parasites, viruses, or whatever. However, in my opinion, if your body is cleansed and healthy, you don't need a laboratory to build you an antibiotic. In 24 to 48 hours, your body will build its own antibodies to take care of the "invaders," and will wipe out the particular disease trying to establish roots in your system.

On the other hand, if you have been feeding your body only junk food, pre-processed food, preservatives, additives, and food low in nutrients, your body is the proverbial "accident going somewhere to happen." Your immune system will be low to nonexistent, and your body will be easy prey for the first "bug" to come along.

Another condition having now been determined as epidemic in proportion is lumps (tumors—fibroid benign or malignant) in ladies' breasts. In my opinion, lumps in the breast are nothing more than congested lymphatic glands. Of course, if women were getting the right nutrition and their lymphatic system was working properly, along with their immune system, and they were eating correctly and getting the right amount of exercise and rest, there would not be such an epidemic.

Finally, a sad statistic concerns the great number of children under the age of eight who have cancer. Many years ago, this was unheard of. But doctors recently have reported a growing number of young children who have cancer. I believe it takes several years to pollute your body to the point where the cancer can get a foothold. But I believe as a result of the poor diet the mothers of these children are eating during their pregnancy, we are seeing an exploding number of birth defects in this country, as well as infants who haven't got the ability to resist what they should be able to fight off.

If you are considering having a child, you should start thinking about getting ready for the baby long before you think about getting pregnant... that means getting *your own body* ready, not the nursery nor your job schedule nor the babysitter.

When you have a body that is not cleansed, with all the organs functioning well, you will not be able to supply the baby with the things that it needs to build its own body and organs in your womb. This can result in anything from full-blown disease and birth defects, to a weakened immune system and weak organs that can't properly function to protect and defend the newborn child.

Give it some thought... it makes a lot of sense. If you are already pregnant, it is very difficult for you to cleanse, but at the very least you can start giving your body nutritional benefits, which can be passed on to your baby to help it build strong systems so that it won't become one of those sad statistics (developing cancer before age eight).

I heard of a case where a new mother was about to lose her mind because she had a baby who wouldn't stop crying. The baby appeared to be in good health, otherwise, but cried all the time. To give the mother a break to get some sleep, the grandfather came over to tend the new baby.

Seeing the can of nearly empty cola sitting on the table, he was reminded how his daughter drank colas constantly during her pregnancy, and he got an idea. He dipped his finger into the remaining cola and let the baby suck a few drops from the tip of his finger. Within minutes, it turned over and went right to sleep. This mother had given birth to an infant who was hooked on cola . . . actually, it probably was the caffeine and/or sugar in the cola on which he was hooked, but he was hooked, nevertheless, just as surely as if it had been cocaine, crack, or heroin. I'm sure the result would be the same if the mother had conditioned the baby to cigarettes, alcohol, coffee, tea, or hot fudge sundaes in sufficient amounts.

Ladies, if you are considering having a child, please give careful consideration to what I have said. God will hold us responsible for what we do to these litle ones, and some day you will stand before the Lord in judgment for your actions that have a direct bearing upon your children's well-being.

As time draws to a close for this world, we are told in Revelation that (among many other terrors) plagues and pestilence will be poured out upon the earth. If we are entering those last days, and I believe we are, I seriously doubt if mankind will ever find medical remedies for these diseases. For if, indeed, they are "God's plagues," man's menial efforts likely will prove to be an exercise in futility.

That doesn't mean that God doesn't still heal supernaturally. If one calls upon the Lord, He has promised to hear, and the Bible says, "I am the God that healeth thee."

In the meantime, cleanse your temple and give it good nutrition, so that it will function as God designed it . . . with the natural ability to fight off the onslaught of disease, plague, and pestilence.

Conclusion

While reading this book, I know that some of you subconsciously are trying to find an easier way to do this program. That is to be expected. I constantly battled that same thing. . .trying to find an easier way, a better, a faster way, without having to go through some of the things that are mentioned in here.

Be assured, I will continue to search for a better and easier way, but as of today, there is no better or easier way than what is described in this book. Now, there are slower ways to achieve the same end, and you may do it any way you prefer. Just remember that the goal is to cleanse your body inside to the point that it is capable of repairing the damage that you have done it. Then you will find that the body will heal itself. Until it is cleansed enough to heal itself, you will continue to have sickness, aches, pains, and disease.

A lot of you are thinking, "Let me take an herb, let me take a pill, let me change my way of eating." Well, herbs do help in some cases. Normally, they are so slow that they cannot cleanse the body at the speed we need, because we have disobeyed the health laws in God's Word. A lot of you are thinking that you can't fast, because fasting will absolutely devastate you. Not so! That is mostly in your mind, and you will find when you start fasting that it actually will strengthen your body, because most of you are giving up energy and a lot of vital force from your body by eating the wrong foods and too much of the wrong foods. Even eating too much good food destroys the energy, the enzymes, and the life force (the vitamins and minerals) of your body.

Some of you are thinking, "I want to do the program a little at a time." While it is true that you probably took 30 or 40 years to get *unhealthy,* you probably do not have 30 or 40 years left to get *healthy.* If you cleanse correctly, normally speaking, you can cleanse seven years of bad eating and mistreating the body in seven days. Now, that doesn't always hold true, but it is sort of a "rule of thumb" we have discovered that you can use to gauge what it will take for you to get clean and healthy.

Some of you don't want to do the colon irrigation. Well, that's understandable, but if all you want to do is enemas, you'll have to think of it in terms of about 50 enemas a day in order to get enough irrigation through your body to start diluting the toxins and impurities that you have been putting in your it. Of course, the fastest way is using the 703 Cleanse, which really only means seven days of cleansing, using O_3 (which is activated oxygen) to help expedite removal of the toxins.

Now, I know that many of you can come up with all kinds of excuses why you can't do this program, and believe me, I've heard them all—some of the *dumbest* excuses that man ever could create. But if you want a clean body, a clean and yielded vessel, then you will do the program.

Some of you may rebel and not do the program according to this book. You may stumble upon a new and better program, but in that event, I challenge you, please share it with me, and I will put it in the book at the next printing. I am not greedy with my knowledge—I share it freely with everybody. But this is the fastest way that I have found, and people normally are not patient enough to do things slowly, although I am a firm believer that the body likes gentle therapy, a little at a time, rather than the "sledge hammer" approach.

We have become a society of instant gratification . . . we want what we want when we want it, and that's *right now!* Of course, I understand that. That's the reason this program was developed— to get the best possible program, in the shortest length of time, with the least amount of energy and effort on our part.

Some of you will say you can't afford to buy the

Colema Board or Colonic Board. That's o.k. Find a friend who has a talent to cut up some wood and make you one to go on your toilet. A lot of you say you can't afford to buy the activated oxygen machine to put the oxygen in the water to enable you to cleanse fast. That's o.k. Use enemas. Use whatever means it takes, but start cleaning up your body.

There are people in some of the former Communist countries who are undertaking cleansing that is far harsher than you will ever consider. They are having to build their own boards, heat the water in the house in the winter time, take it outside, and do their cleansing in an outdoor toilet. But they are getting healthy. They have no money to buy the ingredients, so they are using the herbs of their land in the water to purify their systems, and it still works, because when you cleanse the body correctly—from inside—then you will be healthier and better able to be used by God for His service.

Now, if those who profess to be our teachers in divine matters would set a proper example, as well as teach us how to preserve our bodies in good health, they would do much to make the road to heaven easier. People need to be taught that a well-ordered life and strict temperance is the path to health for both the body and the mind, and that only when the body and mind are healthy can God's purpose in our lives be fulfilled.

I believe that each person is a cell in the body of Christ, and if your cell is unclean, you will not help the cell next to you, because you are contaminated. You only can tear down the cell next to you, so that neither can work efficiently. But when you are cleansed inside physically of toxins and inside spiritually of those things not pleasing to the Lord, you will no longer contaminate the cell next door, and you each will begin building the body of Christ.

When we all cleanse, then we can be like a beautiful orchestra, with all the body's cells, organs, and glands working in harmony to make beautiful music for our Lord and Savior.

Let me give you one final admonition. Like anything else in our lives that doesn't receive the proper priority, cleansing and diet can become an idol. There are many people who live their lives on the premise that if a little bit is good, a lot is better (when, in fact, sometimes too much is dangerous). They have enjoyed such terrific benefits from cleansing, that they now are beginning to "overindulge," for lack of a better word—all they think about is what they are going to eat and drink, and how soon they can do their next cleanse. God never intended our body to receive so much of our time and attention that it becomes an idol. Remember, in the New Testament we are told that all things are lawful for us, though not all things are expedient (good for us), and this was referring to eating habits. Then in the same context, we are told not to condemn another brother if his conscience won't let him do what doesn't bother us at all, and don't offend him or be a stumbling block to him.

So, cleanse your body and nourish it properly, but don't go so far that you actually are worshiping the temple instead of the One Who occupies it.

We ask all this in Jesus' name...Amen.

Technical Information For Doctors and Health Practitioners

Ozone—What Is It and What Are Its Benefits?

We hear an awfully lot about ozone these days, but do we actually know what it is? Most of us, I am confident, do not! So to better understand ozone (sometimes referred to as activated oxygen), how it functions, and its benefits to us, we are going to eavesdrop on an interview that will answer these questions for us. We will just label the speakers on the following transcript as Speaker 1 (S-1:), the interviewer, and Speaker 2 (S-2:), the scientist. Now, let's learn about ozone.

S-1: Well, tell me, what is ozone?

S-2: Let me think of an easy way to put this.

O.K., you know what oxygen is. . . you take two atoms of oxygen stick them together, and that's what you breathe every day—O_2. If you take the same atmospheric oxygen, which we all breathe every day, and you pass it through an electrical spark, or if you pass it through an energy field of shortwave ultraviolet light of 254 nanometers, those two atoms come apart and are recombined into three atoms. So what you have in ozone is oxygen with three atoms stuck together instead of two.

S-1:   So that's three atoms of oxygen.

S-2:   Yes sir, that's pure oxygen. But it's a more reactive form of oxygen than regular atmospheric oxygen, because you've put energy into the atoms. You've got three atoms together, and it doesn't want to stay that way. . . it's like a wound-up spring that wants to come undone. Eventually it's going to go back to a single atom of oxygen again in O_2, which is what you breathe.

S-1:   In nature, where do we find it naturally?

S-2:   Well, you've heard about the ozone layer and the alleged problems with the hole in the ozone layer. What is happening is that oxygen floats from the surface of the earth and goes up to the ionosphere; here it meets high levels of ultraviolet energy—shortwave UV energy. That ultraviolet energy is what breaks down the oxygen into two atoms, and it recombines as three, which is ozone. Again, ozone and oxygen are the same thing . . . it is just O_3 instead of O_2. It's the ozone that is up there that absorbs the ultraviolet energy and keeps the shortwaves from coming down here and causing skin cancer.

S-1:   How is some of this ozone beneficial to the earth?

S-2:   Ozone is a natural purifying agent. Ozone, being heavier than air, will eventually float back down to the surface of the earth in very small quantities, and it's the greatest purifier ever known to mankind. It destroys any virus or bacteria in the earth. This is the reason people don't get sick outdoors in the air; they get sick inside of hospitals where you don't have ozone, and you don't have ultraviolet sunlight to sterilize the air. People would never get sick outdoors because of the ozone and the ultraviolet light from the sun. We're talking very, very small quantities to keep the atmosphere sterile. But if it weren't for ozone and ultraviolet light, everybody would be dead on this planet because disease would be prevalent.

S-1:   Is it beneficial to our fruit trees and vegetables?

S-2:   I think it's probably beneficial simply because it keeps them from getting contaminated. You really can't grow produce in a contaminated environment without carrying disease through the food chain to people. So it's important to produce because that's what keeps the environment in which they are growing sterile and free of disease-causing germs.

S-1: Assuming man had not polluted the earth (which we have), and we were the first men on earth, and we happened to have a meter for testing it, we could probably test any river or lake and find them totally pure and high in ozone.

S-2: Well, a stream doesn't have to be high in ozone to be pure; it takes very, very little ozone to purify a stream, .05 parts per million (ppm). So we're talking about small quantities. But if we were to go back a hundred years ago, that's how the water was purified anyway—naturally. There was dissolved oxygen in the water already from rivers going over stones and rapids, and this type of thing, absorbing atmospheric oxygen, and then, of course, you also had sunlight penetrating that water which contains small amounts of ultraviolet light. That converts the oxygen to ozone, and we've talked about that phenomenon. So, when you have O_3 ozone in the water and you have ultraviolet light, the water purifies itself. That's the natural purification agent for cleaning up a river or stream, and if we weren't throwing all those pollutants and contaminants into those streams, they all would be pure.

S-1: What is the negative ion relationship to ozone?

S-2: Ozone is a negative ion because it wants to give up electrons. It is a highly charged molecule. There are all kinds of negative ions; ozone is just one of them.

S-1: We hear about little machines that put negative ions into your room so you will sleep better at night, etc. but what they really are putting into the room is ozone—right?

S-2: Sure, because ozone is also described as a negative ion. This is why people sleep better after a storm. You get lightning and lightning converts oxygen into ozone. When they say there are a lot of negative ions after a storm, it's because there is a lot of ozone, and they are the same thing. But these are *healthy* negative ions.

S-1: Another thing we have heard is that anything that has an "unpaired" atom is considered a free radical. Ozone could be considered a free radical, but it's a good free radical.

S-2: That's right. Another example of a free radical is chlorine, but that is a very destructive toxic free radical and it destroys cells. Ozone is a free radical, but it is quite compatible with the human body, and it doesn't destroy cell tissue.

S-1:   We know you are knowledgeable about the purification of swimming pools and spas, and I'd like to know about the benefits of putting ozone into that water.

S-2:   There are probably two basic ways to sterilize water for pools and spas. One is to put a lot of chlorine in there, which is a very toxic material and creates a lot of chlorine byproducts, which are extremely toxic even as low as 150 parts per billion (ppb). These are THM's, chlorinated biocules that are the byproduct of chlorination.

S-1:   O.K. THM's let talk about that. Can chlorine be linked to cancer, too?

S-2:   In the chlorination process itself, chlorine combines with natural organic matter, decaying vegetation, to form potent, cancer-causing trihalomethanes (THM's) or haloforms. Trihalomethanes collectively include such carcinogens as chloroforms, bromoforms, carbon tetrachloride, bischlorothane, and others. The amount of THM's in our drinking water theoretically is regulated by the EPA. Although the maximum amount allowed by law is 100 ppb, a 1976 study showed 31 of 112 municipal water systems exceeded this limit.

S-1:   And also in spas?

S-2:   The spa, the swimming pool—they have the same problem as the drinking water.

S-1: We know that your company manufactures the Clean Bath, so could you tell us a little bit about the good features of the Clean Bath.

S-2: The Clean Bath was a later version of another product, and that was one that we made for spa owners who didn't want to have to sit in 4 ppm of chlorine. They were well aware of the fact that you absorb chlorine through the pores, especially at elevated temperatures. They were looking for an alternative, so we made them a Clean Spa, which uses ozone to sterilize and purify the water, so they don't have to use chlorine. It came to my attention that a lot of people who don't own spas still wanted the therapeutic effects of using the ozone, so we modified the product so that anybody could use it in a bathtub and ozonate the water, clean it up and purify it, and then sit in there with the Oxygen-Plus floating dispenser in a safe, high oxygen content. By the way, so far as we know, this is the only ozone generator that injects activated oxygen into the water for colonics, spas, and baths, that is manufactured in full compliance with federal standards and is legal in every way.

S-1: We also asked you to develop another product, which was the Oxygen Plus.

S-2: Well, basically, the Oxygen Plus is a large water container, either a one-gallon size or a five-gallon size. It is a plastic container that will not leach any chemicals into the water. You fill it up with water. It has a spigot in it. It has an ozone converter, so while you are using it you don't get excess ozone into the environment where you will breathe it. But it was designed to ozonate water. In addition to bathing, it may also be used to cleanse produce. We know that people handle the stuff many different times. To decontaminate it, put the produce into this container, fill it up with water, and ozonate it for perhaps 20 minutes. This would break down any herbicide or pesticide residuals, plus you would disinfect the produce, killing any virus or bacteria formations on it, and just in general clean it before you consume it.

S-1:   Which is much better for you; you're not putting that virus into your body when you are eating the products that are truly clean. Last, of course, is the drinking water. You actually can use the Oxygen Plus for making drinking water from tap water?

S-2:   Well, that product really is designed to use water that already has been purified and cleaned by a water purification system. But the one-gallon unit was designed to increase the levels of ozone and oxygen in the clean water. Many people feel that there are a lot of benefits from drinking it.

S-1:   So, drinking the ozonated water puts more oxygen into the bloodstream.

S-2: Well, that's the idea.

S-1: We know that you also have developed the Ultra-Sun Water Purification System. Could you tell us about that?

S-2: I think everybody has a need for an easy-to-use home water purification system. The bottled water industry has grown by a billion dollars a year, so the public is becoming well aware of the fact that tap water needs some improvements. We took a look at water purification systems, and none of them address microbiological issues. They all are designed to remove chemcials. Ours is designed to remove chemicals, filter out particulate matter (dirt) from the water, and clean it up. But the unique thing about the Sun-Pure Water Purification System is that it not only removes the chemicals, but it is also a microbiotic water purifier. Basically, all water is contaminated to some degree. A study just released by *Water Technology Magazine,* has pointed out that treated chlorinated tap water may well be contaminated by a virus, as well as bacteria. You cannot filter these things out with a filter alone. You cannot remove them with a reverse osmosis membrane, because they go through membranes—a virus is too small, they pass right through. So, you must treat them with ultraviolet light, just as occurs outside in nature in the natural process. But by radiating the water with UV light, you sterilize it. What our product does is remove the chemicals from the water first, then sterilize it. It is both a chemical purifier and a microbiological purifier. It is easy to use and easy to install.

S-1: And it doesn't cost much per year to run it?

S-2: No, as a matter of fact, you will need a Replacement Kit only about every twelve to fourteen months. The Replacement Kit is very reasonably priced and replaces the three modular components. This can be done in minutes by removing one screw. That's good for about 1,400 gallons of water, and the cost works out to about 5¢ a gallon.

S-1: I am reminded of the incident at the Olympics in Los Angeles when the European Olympic athletes refused to swim in our Olympic pool because it was chlorinated. I understand they had to make one of the pools an ozonated purification system.

S-2: Well, the Olympic-sized pool at UCLA was converted to ozone. They used absolutely no chlorine whatsoever. You already stated the reason why. The European folks won't swim in chlorinated water. They know it's not healthy. It's hard on the eyes and hair, and it probably has a lot of other problems that are not well understood, but that pool is operated entirely on ozone, with no chlorine at all. They've been doing that for three years, now.

S-1: You asked me to read for background information a book by Joseph M. Price, M.D., *Coronaries/Cholesterol/Chlorine.* Maybe you would like to address some of the good reasons people should read this book.

S-2: Dr. Price wrote this book about ten years ago. He was the first person to realize that chlorine in tap water created an awfully lot of serious health problems. He had a theory that the chlorine would raise the cholesterol levels in the water and contribute to heart attacks, strokes, arthritis, and these types of things. That was a time when such a theory was not a popular thing to believe. But he did an animal study on chickens—500 chickens divided into two groups. To one group he gave tap water with half of one ppm, and the other half drank unchlorinated water. He proved, after four or five months, that the animals that drank the chlorinated water developed hardening of the arteries, deposits began to build up inside the artery walls, they suffered strokes, they suffered heart attacks. The EPA did a similar study just three or four years ago on pigeons, and arrived at the exact same results that Dr. Price discovered.

S-1: I think it would be a "must" for people to read this book. To locate it, request it by the title and ISBN No. 0-515-09461-7. It costs only $2.95, and I'll furnish the address at the back of the book so people can buy it.

S-2: I think reading that book can change a

person's way of life.

S-1: Can you think of any other literature you would like to recommend on ozone and chlorine, that would make people's lives simpler?

S-2: There are volumes and volumes of material available on this subject. Much of it is in the public library. . .you could study there for months and months and not run out.

S-1: Do you think the average water purification system in the average city in the United States is adequate?

S-2: Well, I don't know what average is, and, again my concern for the filtration systems is that they can only filter out the larger particles and chemicals; they can do nothing to purify the water from biological entities. And it is a well-known fact that filters are a breeding ground for bacteria, unless you have an ultraviolet system to destroy them. So if you are filtering, you probably are decreasing particles and chemicals, but increasing bacteria. It's kind of a toss-up which is worse. You really need a system that includes passing the water through ultraviolet treatment to have truly clean water.

That concludes our interview.

Hydrogen Peroxide and Its Uses

I first was introduced to hydrogen peroxide, which is H_2O_2, by listening to a lecture given by a man named Walter Grotz at the National Health Federation. He also had somebody else on the platform by the name of Father Wilhelm.

He told me a story about how he was working with some of the elderly people in some of the retirement homes, and how they were having some problems with certain diseases, and how a man from the Mayo Clinic by the name of C. E. Rosenow came down to the clinic in the southern state and was able to isolate the particular disease that was causing the problem. While he was there, Father Wilhelm complained about having some stiffness in his joints, and Rosenow told him that if he would drink a simple solution of hydrogen peroxide this problem would go away. He gave him the formula and Father Wilhelm tried it—it worked! Within a few weeks his problem went away, so he shared with other people, like Walter Grotz, and Walter Grotz went out in the world and started lecturing on it.

I'd like to praise all three of the people for their part in the evolution of this oxygen therapy. While Grotz' method worked, many people have developed other types of hydrogen peroxide products, some in a powder form, some in a liquid form that they put in drinks, and a variety of other ways for using hydrogen peroxide. I used it myself for about four years. I found it to be excellent because it did increase my health and made my life better, but it's a very unpleasant product to drink.

I want to clarify something. What they told me was to make sure that I had "food grade" hydrogen peroxide, and not the stuff off the shelf in the local drug store. The formula recommended was a simple solution; have a very diluted drink three times a day, and then gradually increase it until you get up to the strength that your body can stand. I found that many people, in doing this, got rid of several types of discomfort.

I also was watching the same stuff being used at many of the clinics in Mexico, and they were using it beyond just the drinks. They were using hydrogen peroxide in spas, they were using it in water in which the people would soak, the bath, they were using it to clean their vegetables and fruits, in fact, many of them were using an IV drip of diluted hydrogen peroxide—very much diluted —and there are many doctors around the world who are doing this right now. It goes into the veins through IV drip.

In watching some of the people using hydrogen peroxide products, I noticed the minute they stopped using some of the products, that within a few months, some of their original aches and pains came back. So what that told me was that in order to maintain, they had to stay on the hydrogen peroxide for quite a while, maybe the rest of their lives. The reason is that they were not solving the problem . . . they were only applying hydrogen peroxide to alleviate the symptoms.

Other Forms of Oxygen Usage

In watching some of these alternative clinics, I saw them using activated oxygen (ozone) in many forms. In most cases, they would take the blood out—just like when you donate blood—and mix it immediately with activated oxygen. It would turn to a brilliant pink, then they would drip that same blood right back into the same patient. You could actually see an increase in the live blood analysis of the oxygen content of the blood within 30 minutes.

We saw other people who were doing what they call autohemotherapy, which was taking the activated oxygen and inserting it right into the vein. You would think that because the activated oxygen (ozone) is a gas, it immediately would kill the patient, but it didn't. They very slowly were administering up to 120cc of activated oxygen into a patient until they experienced discomfort in the lungs. When the discomfort started, they stopped the IV. It would give the patient a little discomfort in the lungs and in the lung cavity. But I was amazed at how they were able to actually put gas right into the bloodstream and not hurt anybody.

Many other people were administering activated oxygen (ozone) into the chelation packet at the end of the IV drip toward the end of the chelation therapy to give the body an oxygen boost. I watched and saw many other clinics that were using activated oxygen.

They were doing what they called vaginal and

rectal insufflation, which means they were inflating those two organs with the ozone gas that was being produced through medical oxygen. They were doing maybe 30 seconds of insufflation, maybe as many as half a dozen times a day or more. I thought this was just another way of getting oxygen to the body, but I found out they had some problems. I ran into some people who, in doing that, thought that if two or three is good for you, they want to do a dozen, and if a dozen is good, they want to do two dozen. . .people are impatient.

What happened was that they were oxidizing some heavy metals in their body, which they didn't know were there. One particular lady had had a hair analysis, which told her the amount of chemicals in her body, and the copper content in her body registered normal. But when she started using the insullations, she felt bad, and she actually wound up bedfast. So she ran another hair analysis, sending her sample to the lab in Arizona. When the results came back, she had gone five times off the scale, which means that she had oxidized copper that she didn't know she had at the body tissue level, and now it was being circulated throughout the whole body, and she *really* felt bad. Of course, the body eventually took care of that, and she got better. But because of that, I am very hesitant about doing vaginal or rectal insullations.

This treatment has come under some tough scrutiny recently, because of injury to many people, primarily because of misuse. I do not recommend it because there are safer and more effective methods available to supply the needed oxygen to the blood.

I decided to get involved in the building of a reasonably priced ozone machine—the ones available at the time cost between $8,000 and $20,000. Most of them were from Germany and those particular machines cost more than I wanted to spend, so I went to a company in Orange County, California, from which I had purchased a water system, and I asked if they could develop an inexpensive ozone machine that we could use for doing some of these programs. In spending a lot of money with him . . . and a lot of talking . . . and some more money, finally he came up with a product.

The end result was an ozone machine—not as good as the ones you're using through a corona discharge, because it won't make the heavy concentration. But it makes a concentration of ozone that is pleasant to the body, because using UV to produce ozone (instead of the corona discharge), there is no worry about producing any nitrates or other harmful gases (unless you have very polluted air going into the machine). Since we always use the air inside our home, it usually is not that polluted. No one has every been hurt, nor have we ever had any ill-effects personally.

As you may have determined, I was my own guinea pig in these experiments. We were doing the ozone in the baths. One of the requirements given to this company was to produce an ozone machine that we could use in the bath and spa without being in violation of any federal standards. EPA has a standard, and OSHA enforces it. I understand the standard is: if you smell ozone, it is already five times stronger than it should be. Now, in some of the room humidifiers and purifiers that produce ozone, you can actually smell the ozone coming out. I find the smell of that particular ozone to be objectionable, but I do use it occasionally in our home, especially when we want to make the air smell nice and sweet. If we are going to be gone a day or two, we turn it on and let it purify the air in our house while we are gone—we do not run it continuously while we are there.

Therefore, the ozone machine was designed to produce ozone to put into the bath water or spa, but not put any ozone in the air, so you couldn't breathe anything harmful to you. I do believe that if ozone is strong enough, it can and will affect the membranes of the lungs and nose. I never have had a problem, and I've breathed an awfully lot of ozone, going into the rooms where I'm producing it for myself, but I try to limit myself to being in a room not more than 15 to 20 minutes if the room has ozone being pumped into it. I certainly wouldn't shut the door and leave it on all night in a room I was going to occupy. I find nothing wrong with what I'm doing, but be your own judge and be careful about what you're doing. Again, use your common sense.

After taking an ozone bath, you could see a difference in the blood. It was very slow, because it sometimes took 30 minutes for it show up. So

I got a bag from the supplier that sells to the morgue...yes, I got me a body bag! I actually put the fittings on the body bag, and I would crawl into that thing, maybe up to my waist, and turn on the ozone machine and pump ozone into the tissue around my body from the waist down. Then I would watch my blood 30 minutes or an hour later and decide what was good for me. Well, it was kind of a "hit and miss" proposition, so I bought an SAO2 meter, which tells you (without piercing the skin) the amount of oxygen saturation of the blood by merely sending two light beams through your finger. You can see an immediate response in the body bag, but it would not tell me the amount of oxygen at the tissue level. It would tell me only the amount of oxygen of the blood that had being circulated through my body. And the first machine cost about $5,000. The next machine I bought was a PO2 meter which cost about $15,000 and it tells you the oxygen at the tissue level.

Now, these are kind of expensive toys, but something that I needed. And I found out that body bag was nice, especially if somebody had a problem with their legs, such as gangrene or something, if the doctor would put that particular patient into a hypervaric chamber and pressurize it with 2 to 2½ atmospheres of oxygen, that usually it prevented the need for amputation. I found out that some people who had poor circulation and poor oxygen content in their extremities could benefit from a body bag, or just a leg bag, of the ozone. But it was still a "hit and miss" proposition.

We got into doing baths in a bathtub or a spa. We found that during an hour bath, where you are actually pumping ozone into the water, that all the excess ozone that the water didn't take would be converted back to O_2. So, you were only breathing O_2, which is what you normally breathe anyway, but all the O_3 that went into the water was oxygen available for the body, to be absorbed through the skin. I understand that .1 ppm (parts per million) is the maximum you can pump into the water, and you're trying to compete with the oxygen that's already in the water, so that's about the maximum that anybody can pump into water and make the water accept.

We found that by taking a soaking for an hour in the bath of ozone water, or in a spa, and scrub the skin three times in that hour, we could put as much oxygen into our blood and into the tissue level of the body as we could by the other methods described earlier. And it's a much safer, gentler way of getting oxygen into the body.

Another thing I discovered is that if oxygen gets into the joints and into the tissue level of the body —for example, you had an ache in the knee and it had been there from football practice, or a football injury, and it constantly gave you a little discomfort—the minute we got oxygen into that knee, the pain and aches went away. So really, what we are saying in some cases is that the body is struggling, and any time you have pain, you have a lack of oxygen. That may not hold true throughout the whole body, but in many of the things we experienced, it did hold true.

So, all these are ways of getting your body a greater amount of oxygen, but we found some added beneficial side effects from the bath or spa —the skin became cleaner, it became softer, and it felt like it was alive. Now, occasionally, I would pull the hose off of the floating probe in the bathtub or spa. Y have an ozone generator that sits on the floor and plugs into a 110V and has a plastic hose that goes over the side of the bathtub or spa with a floating saucer that goes in the bathtub or spa; that's what actually produces the ozone in the bath. I would pull the hose off occasionally for maybe 10 or 15 minutes and let some of the ozone into the room where I was bathing. I would be very careful about how much ozone I would breathe, because I didn't want to get real strong ozone and injure the nose or lung membranes. However, I found out that my lungs became cleaner, and if it felt like I was coming down with a little bit of sore throat or a little stuffed up head, while I was in the bath or spa I would breathe a little bit of the ozone. I found that it helped to rid my lungs, throat, and nose of some of the mucus.

Available Helps and Where to Locate Them

To make it easy for you to find helpful materials and supplies, as well as publications referenced in this book, I have listed them in this Appendix. On the following pages you will find a "shopping list" so you will know what to buy before you begin the 703 Cleanse, what you will need if you wish to prepare your own kits (available to health practitioners and health food stores only), as well as additional information on specific products and where they may be purchased.

Hair Analysis

The Eck Institute
8650 North 22nd Avenue
Phoenix, AZ 85021
(602) 995-1581
Call for complete instructions before taking a sample of hair for submission for analysis.

Laboratory Testing

Great Smokies Diagnostic Laboratory
18-A Regent Park Boulevard
Asheville, NC 28806
1-800-522-4762
All test results include detailed interpretation and commentary. Testing is available for: Digestive Analysis, Intestinal Permeability, Parasitology, Microbiology/Mycology Analysis, Immune Function, Cardiac Profiles, and Osteoporosis Risk Evaluation. Inquire about insurance coverage and Medicare.

Recommended Books

Healthy Water
By Martin Fox, Ph.D.
Available from Healthy Water Research,
P. O. Box 173, Portsmouth, NH 03802-0173
Coronaries/Cholesterol/Chlorine
(ISBN 0-515-09461-7

By Joseph M. Price, M.D.
Available from Berkley Publishing Group
390 Murray Hill Pkwy., Dept. B
East Rutherford, NJ 07073
Tissue Cleansing Through Bowel Management
By Bernard Jensen, D.C.
Available from Bernard Jensen Enterprises
24360 Old Wagon Road, Escondido, CA 92027

Your local health food store frequently will have these publications available.

Cleansing Programs

Linda Getty offers cleansing programs for those who need assistance. See complete details on page 235.

Cleansing Kits

Pat Lee has available kits with everything you need to go on the cleanse by yourself. See complete details on page 235. (He also stocks books.)

Cleansing Equipment

Colon boards are available from General Products (see page 239 for details) and Ultimate Trends (see page 238 for details). Oxygenating equipment, Oxy-Plus container, and water purifiers are available from Ultra-Sun Technologies (see pages 236 and 237 for details and descriptions).

The Shopping List

You will need to buy the following items before you can begin your 703 Cleanse Program (on the following pages I have listed some sources where they may be obtained):

Colon Board (colema or colonic board)
Clean Bath (Ozone float device)
Oxy-Plus Container (in lieu of bucket)
Kit/Supplements

Plus the following items from your local health food store:

apple juice
apple cider vinegar
raw unfiltered honey
Hidden Valley Seasoning Broth
cascara sagrada
D.D.S. #1 Lactobacillus Acidophilus

Assembling Your Own Kits

(Available only to health professionals or health food stores.)

Available from Bio-Energy Systems, Inc., 1-800-858-4160
Enzymes 321A, 649A, and L. Salivarius

Information only: Cyanotech Corp (808)
Orders only: Pat Lee 1-800-888-1374
Spirulina Pacifica

Information only: Bio-Guard Plus 1-800-888-6693
Orders only: Pat Lee 1-800-888-1374
Superoxide Dismutase (S.O.D.)

Available from health food stores
Vitamin C, Niacin, Beet tablets or crystals, Dulse, Flax seed oil, Sonne #7 and #9, Calphonite, D.D.S. #1 Lactobacillus Acidophilus, and Vitamin/Mineral Supplement.

Colon Cleansing Kits

Pat Lee has helped hundreds of people through the 703 Cleanse Program and is willing to answer any questions you may have. You may call him with inquiries at (303) 495-0995 from 3:00 to 6:00 p.m., Mountain Time, Monday through Friday. (The 800 number listed below is only for placing orders.)

Complete Colon Cleansing Kit includes: Ozone Machine, Oxy-Plus Container, Colon Board, all Supplements, Enzymes, and L. salivarius. Supplements are available by the item for use in future cleansing. If you mention this book when ordering, you will receive a substantial discount (discounts apply only to complete kits). He stocks many helpful books, as well.

To Order, call Pat Lee at 1-800-888-1374

Colon Cleansing Programs

Linda Getty operates the Ultimate Tissue Cleansing (UTC) Program. Her staff assists different groups at different places weekly. They use the procedures recommended in this book, including the 703 Cleanse. Maximum results are achieved using state-of-the-art techniques and equipment. She offers a week-long program for those who desire assistance in their personal cleansing. She is available for inquiries at (619) 722-4764, 3:00 to 6:00 p.m., Pacific Time, Monday through Friday.

For information about date and location of the next UTC Program, call, write, or fax: Linda Getty 400 N. The Strand #5, Oceanside, CA 92054-1937 Phone (619) 722-4764; Fax (619) 724-5527.

ULTRA-SUN TECHNOLOGIES, INC.

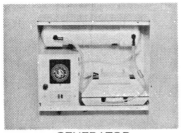

GENERATOR

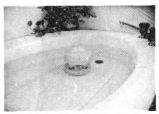

OZONE DISPENSER

Microzone Cleanbath Generator
With Ozone Dispenser
Complete for Bath or Spa

Retail Price $795.00
Special Discounted Price $675.00
  (with photocopy of this page)
UPS Shipping & Handling .... $ 15.00

— OR —

Microzone Cleanbath Generator
With Oxy-Plus 5-Gallon Container
At Same Special Price of $675.00 (Plus Shpg.)

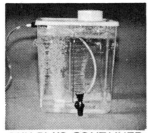

OXY-PLUS CONTAINER

Oxygen-Plus 5-Gallon Activator/Container

Retail Price $187.00
Discounted Price. $ 95.00
  (w/photocopy of this page)
UPS Shpg. & Hdlg... $ 5.00

ULTRA-SUN TECHNOLOGIES, INC.

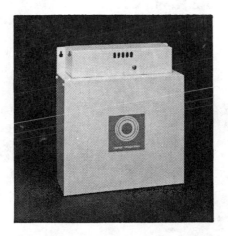

Ultra-Sun Water Purifier

(Specifiy "over" or "under" the counter model)

Retail Price $385.00
Special Discounted Price $325.00
    (with photocopy of this page)
UPS Shipping & Handling .... $ 10.00

VISA and MasterCard accepted. To receive discounted prices, enclose a photocopy of these pages with your order.

Mail Order To:

ULTRA-SUN TECHNOLOGIES, INC.
22342 La Palma Avenue, Bldg. 117
Yorba Linda, CA 92686
(714) 692-1232

Ultimate Home Colonic Unit Model 400
$250.00 + UPS Shipping & Handling
Complete with Bucket

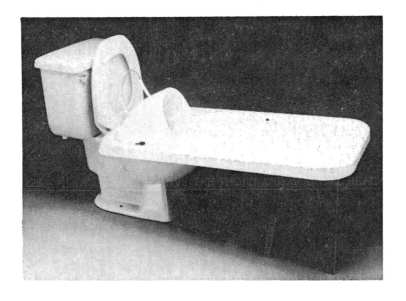

Mail Order To:

ULTIMATE TRENDS, INC.
7835 South 1300 East
Sandy, UT 84094
1-800-745-3191 or (801) 566-3191

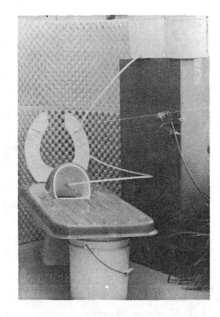

Colema Board
Complete with
Bucket, Hose,
Fittings, and Clamps.
No assembly required.

Retail Price $139.00
Special Discounted Price $125.00
   (with photocopy of this page)
UPS Shipping & Handling . . . . . $ 10.00
   (allow two weeks for delivery)

Mail Order To:

GENERAL PRODUCTS
29426 San Jacinto St.
Perris, CA 92571
Phone (909) 657-2415 / Fax (619) 966-1065

REMOVE THE THORN
AND
GOD WILL HEAL

Additional copies of this book may be obtained from Belco. Please inquire by mail concerning current prices, quantity purchase discounts, or bookstore/trade discounts.

BELCO
10802 S. La Serna Drive
Whittier, CA 90604